Including Students With Severe Disabilities in Schools

FOSTERING COMMUNICATION,
INTERACTION, AND PARTICIPATION

School-Age Children Series

Series Editor
Nickola Wolf Nelson, Ph.D.

Children of Prenatal Substance Abuse
Shirley N. Sparks, M.S.

What We Call Smart: Literacy and Intelligence
Lynda Miller, Ph.D.

Whole Language Intervention for School-Age Children
Janet Norris, Ph.D., and Paul Hoffman, Ph.D.

School Discourse Problems, Second Edition
Danielle Newberry Ripich, Ph.D., and Nancy A. Creaghead, Ph.D.

Including Students with Severe Disabilities in Schools:
Fostering Communication, Interaction, and Participation
Stephen N. Calculator, Ph.D., and Cheryl M. Jorgensen, Ph.D.

Including Students With Severe Disabilities in Schools

FOSTERING COMMUNICATION, INTERACTION, AND PARTICIPATION

EDITED BY:

Stephen N. Calculator, Ph.D., Cheryl M. Jorgensen, Ph.D.

University of New Hampshire
Durham, New Hampshire

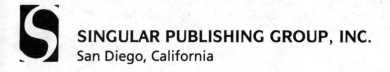

SINGULAR PUBLISHING GROUP, INC.
San Diego, California

Singular Publishing Group, Inc.
4284 41st Street
San Diego, California 92105-1197

© **1994 by Singular Publishing Group, Inc.**

Typeset in 10/12 Palatino by ExecuStaff
Printed in the United States of America by BookCrafters

Library of Congress Cataloging-in-Publication Data

Calculator, Stephen N., 1952–
   Including students with severe disabilities in school : fostering communication, interaction, and participation / Stephen N. Calculator and Cheryl M. Jorgensen (eds.).
     p. cm.—(School-age children series)
   Includes bibliographical references and index.
   ISBN 1-56593-080-0
   1. Mainstreaming in education—United States.
2. Handicapped—Education—United States. 3. Speech therapy for children—United States. 4. Communication in education—United States. I. Jorgensen, Cheryl M. II. Title. III. Series.
LC4031.C19 1994
371.9'046—dc20   94-10002
                                                   CIP

Contents

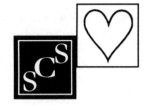

Foreword

Conversations about "inclusion" of children with severe disabilities in today's schools may be complex and challenging, but never boring. As school districts across the western hemisphere have attempted to bring more such children home to their neighborhood schools to be educated in classrooms with their normal learning peers, the topic of inclusion has become familiar to much of the general population. Although the conversations that result are lively and spirited, at times they are more heated by passion than enlightened by information.

It was the passion and vision of a relatively small number of parents and professional advocates that led inclusion to be tried in the first place. They were the pioneers. The civil rights challenge was picked up by others, and the movement spread. However, it was the hard work and dedication of a much larger group of individuals, including parents, teachers, administrators, specialists from a variety of disciplines, not to mention kids, that fostered the development of concepts and strategies for implementing inclusion on a day-to-day basis.

Critics of inclusion also enter the conversation. They express concern about children being plunked down in classrooms and left to stare. They worry about time demands on teachers, distractions to other students, and the possibility that this may represent a return to an earlier time when children with special needs sat in the back of the room working puzzles or coloring ditto worksheets.

Both those who carry the vision and those who worry about it will find *Including Students with Severe Disabilities in Schools: Fostering Communication, Interaction, and Participation* important reading. In writing it, Calculator and Jorgensen gave form to the vision and concrete answers to the critics. In their original pioneering efforts and their continued consulting work as the movement has advanced, the authors have worked through some of the problems the critics worry about first hand. Their liberal use of case examples gets beyond the message of what should be done and begins to address how to make it happen. Suggestions at the program planning level as well as the classroom level help the reader begin to visualize the possibilities for a different way of viewing integration and participation as part of a wider system of communication. The chapter on transitions to adult living by Powers and Sowers is important for taking the discussion beyond the school-age years.

As series editor, I am delighted to have this book extend the three themes that unify the series: collaboration, the influence of context and culture on children's changing needs across the childhood years, and relevance to meeting children's real-life needs. The discussion of inclusion as guided by Calculator and Jorgensen presents opportunities for readers to extend their understanding of each of these themes. It most surely will fulfill its broader purpose of extending opportunities for individuals with severe disabilities and their friends, as well. It is with that conviction that I introduce the book to you.

Nickola Wolf Nelson, Ph.D.
Series Editor

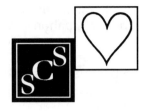

Preface

With the proposed merger of regular and special education, speech-language pathologists (SLPs) and others find their roles changing. This is particularly evident for programs for students with severe disabilities. Although programs once emphasized life skills such as toileting, dressing, eating, and crossing the street, greater emphasis is now placed on academic skills. Skills targeted for instruction are often drawn from regular education curricula and addressed within the context of regular classrooms.

The primary purpose of this book is to provide teachers, SLPs, parents, school psychologists, and others with a vision of how communication and other skills can be taught to students with severe disabilities in regular classrooms and related settings. Communication is not conceptualized as an independent curriculum area nor as a goal in and of itself. Instead, it is presented as a means of enhancing students' active participation in meaningful activities in and out of school, and, as importantly, as a means for developing and maintaining relationships with family and friends.

Within this model, communication gains are not examined through changes in linguistic complexity, vocabulary size, length of messages, and/or ability to access increasingly more sophisticated technological aids (e.g., augmentative communication devices). Instead, these and other variables are subordinated to examination of the role of communication in facilitating students' development and maintenance of friendships, promoting their active participation in classroom routines, and increasing social contacts with peers and others. These indices are consistent with collaborative models of service delivery in which team members' respective contributions reinforce a set of common, mutually agreed on goals and priorities. Communication strategies for elementary and secondary level students are discussed as part of the bigger picture of inclusive schooling.

Students With Severe Disabilities

All students, irrespective of the nature or severity of their disabilities, have equal rights to a free and appropriate public education "in the least restrictive environment (LRE)." It is the authors' contention that, with the proper supports, the least restrictive environment for all students, including those with severe disabilities, can be regular classrooms.

This book focuses on students with severe disabilities, defined by the National Joint Committe for Meeting the Communicative Needs of Persons With Severe Disabilities (1992) as including persons with severe to profound mental retardation, autism, and other disorders that result in severe sociocommunicative and cognitive communication impairments. Although this population is tremendously heterogeneous, previous authors have found similarity among students in their ongoing needs for support in most life activities (Bellamy, 1985). Perhaps Gold (1980) expressed this best stating that, "the height of a person's level of functioning is determined by the availability of training technology and the amount of resources society is willing to allocate and not by significant limitations in biologic potential" (p. 5).

Throughout this book, strategies for identifying and addressing the individual needs of students, in regular classrooms, are presented. It should be pointed out, however, that not all have shared our belief in the viability of such a model of education. For example, Morsink and Lenk (1992) pointed out that, "a classroom with a great range of individual differences and a large number of students is rarely an appropriate placement for students with severe disabilities" (p. 36). They contended that with increasing class sizes, opportunities for student-teacher interaction decrease and students' individual needs cannot be met.

Morsink and Lenk warn that unless more efficient and effective practices evolve, schools will be unable to meet the needs of an ever-increasing population of students with special needs. Without educational change, they foresee schools evolving to a "common mediocre system" (p. 40) and an eventual collapse of special education.

We strongly support the call for educational reforms that stress teacher training and increased levels of collaboration across the blurring lines that have traditionally separated regular and special education (Gartner & Lipsky, 1987). This book stresses collaborative models of service delivery and encourages readers to redefine their roles as educators. Otherwise, we might find ourselves endorsing programs that purport to include students, yet systematically exclude them from the supports they need to function effectively.

Rediscovering General Education Curricula

Mirenda and Calculator (1993) recommended that, "the regular education curriculum should serve as a basis for educational goal setting and longitudinal planning for *all* students" (p. 47). They cited several benefits associated with this strategy. First, the use of regular curricula assures more continuity of instruction than personalized curricula, which may change with changes of the philosophies and preferences of individual educational staff. Also, the use of regular curricula encourages students receiving support from, and interaction with, classmates. Finally, these authors suggested that involving students in regular curricula enhances their self-perceptions and others' perceptions and expectations of them.

As will be pointed out throughout this book, in inclusive classrooms the process of education is at least as important as the content of instruction. SLPs and other special education staff are now being asked to assume roles that are more supportive and consultative (for students and their classmates, parents, teachers, and other staff), with a de-emphasis on direct instruction. Educational activities are concurrently viewed as opportunities to learn and practice social and communication skills. The SLP is now expected to teach or co-teach communication skills, which are expected to enhance students' levels of participation within classes.

Bridging the Gap Between Philosophy and Action

It is our hope that this book will help bridge existing gaps between philosophy and action (McLean, 1993). The successful inclusion of students with severe disabilities in general education requires more than ideas, philosophies, and values. These students often require individualized and highly specialized services and resources in order to benefit fully from inclusive schooling. This book provides readers with procedures through which students can be included *and appropriately educated*. Practices discussed in this book foster *communication, interaction, and participation*, as the title suggests.

Like their classmates, every one of these students can enrich society as a whole. The extent to which their potential contributions are realized will depend on the quality of educational and related services they receive, and the values, vision, and commitment of the people responsible for those services and supports.

■❑ REFERENCES

Bellamy, T. (1985). Severe disability in adulthood. *Newsletter of the Association for Persons with Severe Handicaps, 11,* pp. 1, 6.

Gartner, A., & Lipsky, D. (1987). Beyond special education: Toward a quality system for all students. *Harvard Educational Review, 57,* 367–395.

Gold, M. (1980) *Try another way training manual.* Champaign, IL: Research Press.

McLean, J. (1993). Assuring best practices in communication for children and youth with severe disabilities. *Clinics in Communication Disorders, 3,* 1–6.

Mirenda, P., & Calculator, S. (1993). Enhancing curricula design. *Clinics in Communication Disorders, 3,* 43–58.

Morsink, C., & Lenk, L. (1992). The delivery of special education programs and services. *Remedial and Special Education, 13*(6), 33–43.

National Joint Committee for Meeting the Communicative Needs of Persons with Severe Disabilities. (1992). Guidelines for meeting the communication needs of persons with severe disabilities. *Asha, 34*(3), (Suppl. 7), 1–8.

Contributors

Editors

Stephen N. Calculator, Ph.D., CCC-SLP
Professor
Department of Communication Disorders—Hewitt Hall
University of New Hampshire
Durham, New Hampshire

Cheryl M. Jorgensen, Ph.D.
Project Coordinator and Research Assistant Professor
Institute on Disability/UAP
University of New Hampshire
Durham, New Hampshire

Other Contributors

Beth Dixon
Educational Consultant
Institute on Disability/UAP—University of New Hampshire, and, Office for Training and Educational Innovations
Concord, New Hampshire

Laurie E. Powers, Ph.D.
Associate Director
Hood Center
Dartmouth-Hitchcock Medical Center
Lebanon, New Hampshire

Jo-Ann Sowers, Ph.D.
Project Director
New Hampshire Natural Supports Project
Institute on Disability/UAP
Concord, New Hampshire

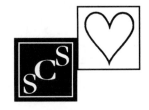

Acknowledgments

We have tried to make this book a useful tool for practitioners rather than an account of research studies conducted with anonymous subjects in a clinical setting. We hope that the personalities of the students described herein emerge as multifaceted as they are in real life. (Note: None of the case studies are fabricated; all involve students who presently attend public schools in New Hampshire and elsewhere.) Without the ongoing collaboration with families and schools that has defined our work, we would not have been able to accomplish these goals. We are grateful for their trust and openness.

We would especially like to thank our own families—Jeannie, Bryant, Lauren, Trevor, and Kaitlin; Neil, Katherine and Anne—for their support and patience. They provide us with daily reminders that inclusion is much more than an educational philosophy concerned primarily with disability—it is an approach to living.

The second author's contributions have been supported in part by a grant from the U.S. Department of Education, Office of Special Education and Rehabilitative Services, Office of Special Education Programs, Division of Innovation and Development, Grant #H023R20018.

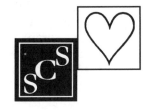

Prologue

Beth Dixon

■□ EMBARKING ON AN UNEXPECTED VOYAGE: ONE PARENT'S VIEW

As the parent of four children who range in age from 10 to 21, there have been many experiences that we have shared and from which we have learned. I would like to focus right now on my youngest child, Andrew, who has led our family through one of our more significant voyages.

When Andrew was born, he was welcomed with the greatest of joy by all of us. He was a beautiful, blonde, blue-eyed, 8 lb 7oz. little boy. My other children sat looking in awe at this little person and talked about how much fun it was going to be to watch him grow, learn to smile, recognize each of us, talk, walk, and so forth. We talked about the cute things babies say when they are learning to express themselves and I related silly, adorable things the older children said when they were babies.

At 7 months of age, we were thrown into a very strange and unfamiliar world of disbelief, of feeling incompetent and power-less. Andrew had been "diagnosed" and our voyage took its first detour. He started in early intervention, and was "provided" therapies (PT, OT, speech) four times a week. We waited and hoped that he would somehow be "fixed" and returned to us as the child we had expected but somehow lost.

Over the next 2 years, I realized that we hadn't lost anything. He was the same beautiful child I had brought home from the hospital. He had the same needs that all children have—to be fed, taken for walks, played with, read to, and loved and cared for by his family and close friends. It no longer mattered that early intervention hadn't "fixed" him. We accepted Andrew for who he was.

Oh, No, School!

Oh no, school at age 3? My other children had played with their friends in the neighborhood and in so doing learned the various social, communicative, and play skills that they needed to interact effectively. The experts knew and I listened as they explained how my son was not "ready" to be with children his age. He would spend 1 hour (each way) on a little yellow bus to attend a $2\frac{1}{2}$ hour readiness program. Here, he would receive intensive one-to-one attention from teachers, aides, therapists, and others. Instruction would take place in a cubby, behind a partition.

At home, we continued to be thrilled with Andrew's accomplishments. Just before he turned 4, Andrew began walking independently. He could now touch and explore all of the things he had previously wanted to, but had been unable to do. He had us running and steering him away from things that could be dangerous. He had such a sparkle in his eyes every time a new opportunity presented itself. I was on guard constantly, but enjoyed watching him explore his newfound world. We thought this was normal, until his teachers began describing him as a child who could not understand danger and whose attention span was nonexistent.

Turning the Corner

Our team requested a consultation from Dr. Stephen Calculator to discuss augmentative communication. Andrew was not speaking yet and it was time to bring in another "expert." I was so nervous that I didn't sleep the night before the assessment. I tried to think of a way that I could get to this man before he heard all of the negatives about Andrew and gave up on my son before even starting.

I did see Dr. Calculator in the hallway as he was on his way to Andrew's classroom. As he approached, all I could think of to say to him was, "Please keep an open mind." I have eaten those words since then. Dr. Calculator looked at Andrew and smiled and Andrew was crazy about him right away.

Together, they tried a basic form of signs and functional gestures. Andrew responded to him. The doctor looked at my child and saw the person I saw—a fascinating 4-year-old boy who, "happened to have some other things going on." For the first time, an expert offered positive observations and comments before launching into recommendations.

Over time, I began to question the wisdom of a program that separated children according to their levels of ability. Whenever I heard about Andrew's lack of imitative skills, my mind screamed, "Who is he supposed to imitate?" Children learn from each other and Andrew wasn't given the opportunity to be with other children from whom he could learn. I asked the team to enroll him in a regular preschool—my suggestion was met with stares of disbelief and a knowing look that this parent was most definitely in denial.

I then attended a series of workshops though the Institute on Disability at the University of New Hampshire, at which state-of-the-art information concerning best practices for children with severe disabilities was presented. As Dr. Cheryl Jorgensen spoke on the topic, "Schools for ALL kids," I felt that she was speaking directly to me. This was the missing piece. Of course Andrew couldn't do what everyone else his age typically does—he didn't know *what* they were doing. He was behind the walls of a cubby.

I then found a local playgroup that Andrew could attend one morning a week. It worked out great. There, he was just another kid. Suddenly, I began receiving different types of reports about my son, "He watched three boys playing with a train set today and, although he didn't join them, he went over to it when they finished and tried to operate it." Aha, imitation skills!

Readiness to be a Child?

We got through preschool, and it was time to enter kindergarten. Big meeting. My husband and I worked out our game plan. He would play the "heavy" as we would attempt to negotiate a regular kindergarten experience for Andrew. The team wasn't ready for such a bold move and so we compromised. Andrew would attend a self-contained program 4 hours a day and would visit the kindergarten each day for a short time. The plan was to gradually extend the amount of time he spent in the kindergarten as he demonstrated an ability to cope in this setting.

One day, I visited the kindergarten to see how Andrew was doing. He arrived a few minutes after me, accompanied by his entire class (from the special program). The teacher greeted the group, "Here come our special friends." I watched the kindergarten children slouch nervously in their chairs. No one interacted with Andrew except the adult who was seated beside him.

This was a turning point for Andrew. We requested a team meeting the following day to express our concerns. Six weeks later, Andrew was included fully in the kindergarten program. His teachers began remarking that Andrew was now looking to his peers for help, rather than to adults. Classmates were now enjoying being with Andrew and helping him.

One day, we were walking around at a local fair when a young girl approached and asked if Andrew could go on a ride with her. He was 5 years old and for the first time was taking a ride with a friend. Unlike my other children, who had gone to dozens of places with their friends by that age, Andrew's attending a school across town had prevented such opportunities from arising. It was time to "come home."

Bringing Andrew Home

At his next IEP meeting, I argued one more time for inclusion. Andrew needed to know how to cross streets, how to play, to communicate with friends . . . to be a kid. We explained that we had no plans to move and that neighborhood children would ultimately be the adults (congressmen, friends, employers, and neighbors) in his future. The decision was made—Andrew would come "home" to Conant School (in our neighborhood) in September!

When his principal, Mr. T., asked me what I most wanted to achieve by including Andrew at Conant School, I replied "I want him to go to a birthday party." Mr. T. replied (with his head in his hands) that he couldn't guarantee that. Two weeks later, I let him know that my goals were met. Andrew was going to a party that weekend.

Speech and OT were part of Andrew's day in the classroom. The therapists would visit and observe what the class was doing and then figure out (with the aide and teacher) how Andrew could participate to his fullest. Where better to learn communication than among 23 peers who were talking all around him? Andrew's attention span was addressed during reading time, as was his need to begin following directions, "Turn the page please." Communication boards were developed and Andrew was now able to make choices, indicate likes and dislikes, and answer questions by pointing to pictures that corresponded to different events and activities.

If You Can't Teach It in a Regular Classroom, Don't Teach It

We continue to struggle with staff who feel that there are things Andrew needs to learn that cannot be taught in his classroom. I have always felt, however, that if a skill could not be taught in the regular classroom, it was most likely something that Andrew would have little use for.

In closing, Andrew's program continues to evolve, as do his family, teachers, aides, and classmates. We all recognize that we are charting territory that was never conceived of at his home school before Andrew and the rest of his family expressed their dreams for inclusive education.

We hope that this book helps the thousands of Andrews who can benefit from inclusive education. The potential to make dreams happen exists, as do the strategies for making dreams realities.

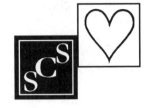

Introduction

Stephen N. Calculator

■□ INCLUSION: IT'S MORE THAN JUST BEING THERE

In the last 20 years, there has been increasing support for and implementation of inclusive practices of education. Stainback and Stainback (1990) defined the inclusive school as one in which all students are educated in the mainstream (i.e., in regular education and regular classes). In an inclusive school, all students' individual needs are met in supportive classrooms. When working properly, inclusive classrooms are places in which students receive appropriate and challenging educational programs that are geared to their capabilities and needs. Support and assistance is available to them (and their teachers) to assure success in the mainstream.

Outcomes of Inclusion

When disagreements about the merits of inclusion arise, they are typically related to questions about whether students with severe disabilities learn more effectively in such settings than in self-contained classrooms, resource rooms, and other specialized environments. Numerous positive outcomes have been associated with the amount of time and frequency of interactions students with severe disabilities have with typical students.

Students who have been integrated in regular education classes have been found to be more likely to participate in other integrated environments in the future (Brown et al., 1987, 1985; Sailor & Halvorson, 1986; Voeltz, 1984); to exhibit more appropriate social behaviors (Falvey, 1980; Gaylord-Ross & Pitts-Conway, 1984; Kahan, 1984; Schactilli, 1987); display more positive affect (Dunlap & Koegel, 1980; Park & Goetz, 1985); and engage in more interactions with others (Anderson & Goetz, 1983; Brinker, 1985; Goldstein & Wickstrom, 1986). There is also evidence that more learning (in terms of the number of Individualized Educational Plan [IEP] objectives met) takes place in such settings (Brinker & Thorpe, 1986; Wang & Baker, 1986).

The California Research Institute recently concluded a set of investigations involving over 20 "statewide systems change projects."These investigations were funded by the U.S. Department of Education to evaluate the impact of these projects on students, families, and schools. Preliminary results indicate that students in inclusive classrooms (regular classrooms in regular education) fared better on several measures pertinent to communication in comparison with their counterparts in self-contained programs within regular school buildings. Their IEPs were more likely to enlist participation and involvement by peers who were nondisabled. As might be expected, these students in inclusive programs were also found to engage in more reciprocal social interactions with nondisabled peers than their counterparts. The latters' interactions with nondisabled peers tended to be more task-related. (Hunt, Farron-Davis, Beckstead, Curtis, & Goetz, 1993). Collectively, these findings suggest increased numbers of opportunities for communication and social interaction in inclusive settings.

Other investigations have focused on the impact of inclusion on students who are nondisabled (typical). Vandercook et al.'s (1991) review of these studies indicate no differences on standardized tests of math and reading such as the *California Achievement Tests* (1985), the *Gates-MacGinitie* (1978), and the *SRA Survey of Basic Skills* (1978). Vandercook et al. (1991) indicate that anecdotal comments by teachers were overwhelmingly positive when discussing the impact of inclusion on their students identified as typical.

Avoiding the Inclusion Delusion

Although some schools have forged ahead with inclusionary practices, their efforts and enthusiasm have stalled after successfully meeting the initial challenge of placing students in regular classrooms. It is not until they attempt to provide IEPs and delineate specific educational goals and expectations for students with severe disabilities, that the greater challenges of inclusion emerge.

One local coordinator of special education, who prefers to remain anonymous, recently chatted with the first editor about what he described as the "inclusion delusion." He talked about the euphoria associated with seeing students with severe disabilities in regular classrooms for the first time. He also talked about his and others' failures to anticipate the amount of work that would then be necessary to assure these students (and their families) that students' educational needs could be met in these same settings.

During the past 8 years, the authors have collaborated with school districts throughout New Hampshire and nationally that have moved toward inclusive schooling. For those districts, the idea that inclusion is attained with little effort is a delusion. The staffs are dedicated people who have persevered through staff identity crises, reassessments of personal and school philosophies, reallocation of resources, and so forth. What began as an attempt to develop an appropriate educational program for a couple of students eventually led to broad changes in school and even system-wide practices. These individuals often discuss how their attempts to include students with severe disabilities have precipitated practices (e.g., delivery of related services in classrooms, increased collaboration between regular and special educators, increased involvement of families, more individualization of curricula, more efficient use of resources) that have benefitted **all** students.

■ WHAT INCLUSION ISN'T

This book posits that inclusive education does not mean that childrens' individual differences be masked or glossed over. A student in an inclusive classroom has not only a right to be there, but an expectation that the youngster will receive an appropriate education in that setting. This connotes access to necessary types and levels of support required to prepare students with special needs for adulthood.

In his keynote address at the Second National Symposium on Effective Communication for Children and Youth with Severe Disabilities, held July 10–12, 1992 in McLean, Virginia, James McLean (1993) offered the following advisory:

> Even though our philosophical and political high ground has been most productive in the arenas specific to educational efforts for children and youth with severe disabilities, we should all realize that our deeds do not yet match the promise of our laws or our language. We should all realize, too, that our philosophical holdings and our revised language do not themselves specify how we will attain our values and our educational goals; they primarily set the targets for that process in which we gather and apply our knowledge on behalf of our children.
>
> I think the difference between language and action is a major issue for us here. Our rhetoric is so good, so stirring, so politically correct, so all-encompassing, that I see a real problem in our confusing language with deeds. To my mind, one of the biggest issues we have to fear is that our words are so fearless, and that, in many cases, they are a world apart from our actions. I say this because, too often, I see inclusionary school settings that really don't include, parent involvement that intimidates rather than involves, and the teaching of functional communication skills that would never be used or be useful in real world situations. (pp. 1–2)

Inclusive education implies far more than just "being there." We contend that the resources necessary to successfully include students with severe disabilities in regular classroom settings now exist in most schools. The personnel are available, students and their families are waiting, the process of change has begun. We hope that this book instills confidence in readers that inclusion can represent more than a philosophy; it can also present a framework for educational reform.

■❑ REFERENCES

Anderson, J., & Goetz, L. (1983, November). *Opportunities for social interaction between severely disabled and nondisabled students in segregated and integrated educational settings.* Paper presented at the 10th Annual Conference of the Association for Persons with Severe Handicaps, San Francisco.

Brinker, R. (1985). Interactions between severely mentally retarded students and other students in integrated and segregated public school settings. *American Journal of Mental Deficiency, 89,* 587–594.

Brinker, R., & Thorpe, M. (1986). Features of integrated educational ecologies that predict social behavior among severely mentally retarded and nonretarded students. *American Journal of Mental Deficiency, 91,* 150–159.

Brown, L., Rogan, P., Shiraga, B., Zanella Albright, K., Kessler, K., Bryson, F., VanDeventer, P., & Loomis, R. (1987). *A vocational follow up evaluation of the 1984–1986 Madison Metropolitan School District graduates with severe intellectual disabilities.* Madison: University of Wisconsin and Madison Metropolitan School District.

Brown, L., Shiraga, B., York, J., Solner, A., Albright, K., Rogan, P., McCarthy, E., & Loomis, R. (1985). On integrated work. In L. Brown, B. Shiraga, J. York, A. Solner, K. Albright, P. Rogan, E. McCarthy, & R. Loomis, (Eds.), *Educational programs for students with severe intellectual disabilities* (Vol. 15, pp. 1–16). Madison: University of Wisconsin and Madison Metropolitan School District.

California Achievement Tests. (1985). Monterey, CA: California Test Bureau/McGraw Hill.

Dunlap, G., & Koegel, R. (1980). Motivating autistic children through stimulus change. *Journal of Applied Behavior Analysis, 13,* 619–628.

Falvey, M. (1980). *Changes in academic and social competence of kindergarten and handicapped children as a result of an integrated classroom.* Unpublished doctoral dissertation, University of Wisconsin-Madison.

Gaylord-Ross, R.J., & Pitts-Conway, V. (1984). Social behavior development in integrated secondary autistic programs. In N. Certo, N. Haring, & R. York (Eds.), *Public school integration of the severely handicapped: Rational issues and progressive alternatives* (pp. 197–220). Baltimore: Paul H. Brookes.

Goldstein, H., & Wickstrom, S. (1986). Peer intervention effects on communicative interaction among handicapped and nonhandicapped preschoolers. *Journal of Applied Behavior Analysis, 19,* 209–214.

Hunt, P., Farron-Davis, F., Beckstead, S., Curtis, D., & Goetz, L. (l993). *Evaluating the effects of placement of students with severe disabilities in general education versus special classes.* Unpublished manuscript.

Kahan, E. (1984). Social skills and the disabled child: A guide to appearance. The *Exceptional Parent, 47–48*

MacGinitie, W. (1978). *Gates-MacGinitie Reading Tests.* Boston: Houghton Mifflin.

McLean, J. (1993). Assuring best practices in communication for children and youth with severe disabilities. *Clinics in Communication Disorders, 3,* 1–6.

Naslund, R., Thorpe, L., & Lefever, D. (1978). *SRA Achievement Series.* Chicago: Science Research Associates.

Park, H., & Goetz, L. (1985). *Affect differences between students with severe disabilities in differing educational programs.* Unpublished manuscript.

Schactilli, L. (1987). *The effects of trained and untrained peer tutors on social behavior of severely disabled students.* Unpublished master's thesis, California State University, Department of Special Education, California Research Institute, Hayward.

Sailor, W., & Halvorson, A. (1986). In *California Research Institute Annual Report, Year 4*. San Francisco: San Francisco State University, Department of Special Education, California Research Institute.

Stainback, S., & Stainback, W. (1990). Inclusive schooling. In S. Stainback, & W. Stainback, *Support networks for inclusive schooling* (pp. 3–23). Baltimore: Paul H. Brookes.

Vandercook, T., York, J., Sharpe, M., Knight, J., Salisbury, C., LeRoy, B., & Kozleski, E. (1991). The million dollar question. . . . *Impact,* 4(3). Minneapolis: Institute on Community Integration, University of Minnesota.

Voeltz, L. (1984). Program and curriculum innovations to prepare children for integration. In N. Certo, N. Haring, & R. York (Eds.), *Public school integration of severely handicapped students. Rational issues and progressive alternatives* (pp. 155–184). Baltimore: Paul H. Brookes.

Wang, M., & Baker, E. (1986). Mainstreaming programs: Design features and effects. *Journal of Special Education, 19,* 503–521.

The Evolution of Best Practices in Educating Students with Severe Disabilities

Cheryl M. Jorgensen and Stephen N. Calculator

■□ INTRODUCTION

This chapter describes a 30-year history of societal attitudes and professional practices concerning the education of students with severe disabilities by (a) presenting a chronology of "best educational practices" for students with disabilities including a discussion of factors that have influenced changes in those practices, (b) discussing concomitant changes in communication practices, and (c) offering the reader three present-day scenarios to analyze relative to the program characteristics presented in the first part of the chapter.

History of "Best Educational Practices"

Prior to this century, people with significant disabilities were victims of euthanasia or life-long incarceration in asylums or other institutions. These practices reflected society's belief that people with disabilities were dangerous, that some disabling conditions were contagious, and that people with disabilities must be prevented from procreating so that their disabilities were not transmitted to their children. These institutions were characterized by inhumane conditions, use of frequent punishment and restraint, and the provision of only food and shelter.

Beginning in the early part of the 1900s, a more benevolent atittude began to develop as state and federal laws were enacted to guarantee some measure of care to people who were institutionalized. The earliest standards of practice that were applied to people with severe disabilities were medically oriented. Those standards were based on a philosophy of custodial care (rather than rehabilitation, training, or education) and dealt with health, cleanliness, staff/resident ratios, and safety. There was little thought given to the need to prepare students or adults for less restrictive placements. School-age student residents with severe disabilities grew into adult residents with severe disabilities, and adult residents lived their lives in the institution (Antonak, 1988).

Example of a Program Based on Custodial Care

Joyce Granger, a 40-year-old woman who now works as a receptionist and lives with support in her own apartment describes with a mixture of sadness and anger her 35 years in New Hampshire's state institution. According to Joyce, she and her older sister were left at Laconia State School in the early 1950s by their single mother who felt unable to care for them, especially when it was discovered that both girls had significant cognitive and behavior challenges. A typical day at Laconia for Joyce began early in the morning when she would be awakened to assist in dressing and feeding other residents whose disabilities were more severe than her own. After breakfast in a communal dining room, Joyce and other children were responsible for helping other staff clean the wards. Joyce was never given any formal educational program—the label "trainably mentally retarded" was applied to her—and her days were spent working around the institution or watching television. Punishment was a common occurence for all Laconia residents and it ranged from spanking for young children to restraint and "aversive behavior management" for older children and adults (Joyce Granger [a pseudonym], personal communication, October 1993).

The First Revolution: Custodial Care to Developmental Practice

Then, in the 1960s, primarily as a result of a number of well-publicized exposes and lawsuits on behalf of institutional residents (Blatt & Kaplan, 1966) regulations were changed to include requirements to provide more systematic training and rehabilitation to people in those institutions. Adults in state or private institutions were then given instruction in activities of daily living and prevocational skills. During that time, some professionals began to envision a life outside of the institution for some people with more significant disabilities. Wolfensberger's notion of "normalization" influenced a small group of professionals at universities and in the field, with community-based sheltered work and group home living promoted as "best practices" (Wolfensberger, 1972).

Although not yet expressed, the notion of "least restrictive environment" was developing. A continuum was envisioned, in which some people who were "ready" might move away from the institution and into the community. With this change in vision—in the expectations of professionals and the community—professionals saw the need to teach new and different skills to people for whom community living might be a possibility. This point is the key to understanding the forces that drive the evolution of best practices. Significant changes in best practices are driven primarily by a shift in beliefs about people with severe disabilities. Although scientific research supporting a change in practice sometimes accompanies the change in philosophy, it is not a prerequisite for change.

For the first time, the notion of measuring outcomes of training and rehabilitation services became salient because professionals and community members on the other end of institutional care—the work supervisors and the group home attendants—had a vested interest in the preparedness of their clients. Although people with disabilities hadn't yet found their consumer voice, others (primarily parents) were now speaking for them and demanding some accountability from the professionals who had responsibility for these individuals before their arrival in the community.

Throughout the remainder of the 1960s and into the early 1970s, this trend continued in small steps (Gold, 1980). Experience with adults with severe disabilities who had benefited from training programs led to advocacy from families and educators to provide educational services for children with disabilities. Public Law 94-142 (P.L. 94-142) and related state laws were grounded in the notion that people (especially children) with mental retardation could learn, and thus, could benefit from educational programs and services (PARC, 1971). P.L. 94-142 stated that all handicapped children were entitled to a free and appropriate public education in the least restrictive environment (Education for All Handicapped Children Act, 1975). For the first time, children with significant disabilities could go to school!

When special education services were first mandated by state and federal laws, concerns about quality were narrowly reflected in efforts to achieve compliance with statutory regulations. Local staff and administrators were required to provide data to state and federal officials, such as the total number of students with educational handicaps being served, the percentage of students with each federally identified disability, and the certification of teachers and other staff providing services for students. Programs were deemed effective if they identified the number of students with disabilities projected by population data, if each student's file contained an up-to-date multidisciplinary evaluation, and if parents were happy with the services their sons and daughters received.

Although research on the outcomes of public education were not available for students with severe disabilities, the field nonetheless promoted some accepted practices in program design and evaluation. During the first few years of implementation of P.L. 94-142, practices were guided primarily by the "developmental theory" that students with disabilities needed to progress through each and every developmental stage of learning and maturation before they could progress to a new stage (Brown et al., 1979). This practice with school age children was different from the developing focus on work and community skills for adults with disabilities. People felt that children with disabilities could "catch up" developmentally so that they would be "ready" for some type of work and community living experience after leaving school. Prior to and following instruction, students were evaluated using tests of normal development in various skill areas (intelligence, sensorimotor, communication, social). A higher score following instruction indicated that teaching was effective. No change or a lower score following instruction was attributed to the inability of the student to learn because of the severity of the student's disability or regression due to the progressive nature of the student's medical condition. A visitor to a typical self-contained classroom operating during this period might have observed the following scene.

Example of a Program Based on Developmental Practice

In the Rainbow Connection classroom, 12 students ages 3–21 with severe disabilities were enrolled from six surrounding school districts. The class was located in a public elementary school, a regional cooperative, or a special education school, and was staffed by a teacher, six full-time paraprofessionals, and part-time physical therapist (PT), occupational therapist (OT), and SLP. The students' ages had little to do with how their day progressed. First thing in the morning, all students were "toileted," and they practiced combing their hair and brushing their teeth. The group then ate breakfast together. Therapists worked on oral-motor skills and labeling of food items using sign language or picture boards for the more developmentally advanced students. Following the communal meal, the students were assembled into a circle for greeting, calendar, and songs. All of the songs were at the preschool level, because the staff noted that even 19-year-old Jodie still smiled and clapped to "The Wheels on the Bus."

Communication goals were implemented by prompting students to hand Polaroid photographs to the student depicted in the picture, as if to say "I know who you are and now it's your turn." Following the circle, students were divided into different therapy and work groups. The PT worked with each student every day on neuromotor developmental skills; the SLP had determined each student's "level" and worked with most on cause-and-effect and object permanence; and the teacher and the paraprofessionals used various preschool toys to teach size, counting, colors, and order relationships. With breaks for lunch, naps, and recess, the students rotated throughout each work group until dismissal time. Six different buses took students back to their home communities at the end of the day, and the following morning the routine began all over again.

The Second Revolution: Developmental Practice to Functional Programming

Beginning in 1979 with publication of the landmark article "The Criterion of Ultimate Functioning and Public School Services for Severely Handicapped Students" (Brown, Nietupski, & Hamre-Nietupski, 1976), the field of special education began striving for something different in after-school life for their students; that is, integration into all aspects of community living including paid work, noninstitutional housing, and participation in community recreational activities. Brown et al. were among the first to suggest that community integration and participation could and should be a reasonable expectation for students with severe disabilities and, most importantly, that there were specific characteristics of school programs that were more likely to result in the realization of those expectations. "Quality program indicators" included: (a) education and support services should be longitudinal, beginning at birth and continuing into adulthood; (b) focus on functional skills, defined as a skill that someone else will have to perform if the student doesn't learn to do it; (c) the instructional environment ought to be the one in which the skill will ultimately be performed to minimize generalization difficulties; (d) age-appropriate materials and tasks should be used; (e) social integration with students without disabilities should be provided; and (f) decisions about program effectiveness should be made based on empirical data.

Later, Brown and colleagues developed curriculum domains based on these principles, called Domestic (self-help and activities of daily living), General Community (street crossing, purchasing), Recreation and Leisure (individual and group free-time pursuits and athletics), and Vocational (real work, not sheltered work) (Brown et al., 1979). School programs during these years were advised to throw out all the commercial toys and make-believe stores and get students out into the community. Ford, Johnson, Pumpian, Stengert, and Wheeler (1980) developed checklists of activities that were appropriate in each of the curriculum domains for students of different ages, and school staff felt as if they were finally working on productive skills that students could use in their adult life.

Schools interested in changing from a developmental to a functional curriculum approach usually needed guidelines for changing their programs in such areas as program philosophy, selection of teaching materials, and responsibilities of program staff. One of the earliest examples of these guildines was developed at the University of Vermont (Thousand, 1987). The "Best Practice Guidelines for Students with Intensive Educational Needs" was organized into six topical areas including (a) age-appropriate placement in local public schools, (b) integrated delivery of educational and related services, (c) social integration, (d) curricular expectations, (e) systematic data-based instruction, (f) home-school partnership, and (g) systematic review of educational and related services. Many school districts in Vermont and other states utilized these practices to help them identify topics for staff training and in program development and improvement.

Meyer (1987) grouped the characteristics of best educational practices into a validated checklist which was prudently titled "Program Quality Indicators (PQI): A Checklist of Most Promising Practices in Educational Programs for Students with Severe Disabilities." This checklist was divided into six sections including (a) program philosophy, (b) program design and student opportunities for learning, (c) systematic instruction and performance evaluation, (d) individualized education plan (IEP) development and parent participation, (e) staff development and team collaboration, and (f) facilities and resources.

Changes in Communication Instruction

The shift from a paradigm that was primarily developmental to one which also emphasized functional skills and preparedness to live, work, and play in home communities quickly found its way into the field of communication disorders. Yoder and Calculator (1981) stressed independence as a primary goal of communication intervention. Subsequent investigators highlighted the need to consider developmental skills to identify possible communication modes and to assist in identifying the content and purposes for which communication might be effective. However, whether communication was to be used to enable individuals to express their basic wants and needs and to indicate choices and preferences or to convey more abstract ideas, the goals remained the same—optimizing their levels of participation in meaningful, functional contexts of interaction.

The following example characterizes an exemplary program during the late 1970s and early 1980s.

Example of a Program Based on Functional Skills Programming

Ms. Farrell's Functional Skills Class at Walker Elementary School was comprised of eight students ages 6–11. The students came from several other schools in the district and had disabilities such as Down syndrome, autism, cerebral palsy, and mental retardation. There were five boys and three girls in the program, and the focus was on readying the students for the junior high school functional skills program, which was vocationally oriented. In the morning, some students rotated among three main activities: school jobs; learning the meaning of signs typically encountered in the community such as food names, stores, street signs, and so on; and cooking. The students who might be considered as having moderate disabilities were given instruction in functional reading and math. In the afternoon, students went on community outings to purchase materials for school programs, shadow workers in community businesses, and do housekeeping chores in the staff's or one another's homes.

During this time, related service professionals attempted to integrate instruction in motor and communication skills into the activities the students were doing. There was a growing emphasis on role release and the transdisciplinary model of service provision (Baine & Sobsey, 1983) so teachers and paraprofessionals could carry out therapeutic teaching even in the absence of itinerant related service staff. Each student attended physical education and sometimes music or art with a mainstream class and was invited to their host classroom for school parties. Students had busy days; they learned important, specific job skills, and, if they were fortunate, obtained part-time work on leaving school at age 21.

Although the researchers and faculty who pioneered much of the work during this era were committed to including students with profound disabilities in functional skills instruction with the goal of postschool community integration, many practitioners in the field felt that little progress had been made in identifying best practices for these students (Sailor, Gee, Goetz, & Graham, 1988). Most students with profound disabilities were still enrolled in segregated programs in developmental centers, special schools, or, occasionally, public school buildings. Their programs still consisted primarily of direct therapy with some attempt to effect their partial participation (doing some steps of each task) in functional activities such as cooking, personal care, and work (Baumgart et al., 1982).

Despite the lack of attention to students with profound disabilities, many students with moderate and severe disabilities were becoming visible in their schools and communities. Families had something to aim and hope for (real job, noninstitutional living, participation in community life), and the term "quality of life" began to take shape for society's most vulnerable people.

The Third Revolution: Introduction of Integration Values

The gains made in school and community programs for people with severe disabilities were significant throughout the 1970s and early 1980s, but there was still much room for growth. People willing to take a hard look at outcomes found that many students' out-of-school lives were devoid of real friendships and community involvement, that adults with severe disabilities were grossly underemployed, and that most people still lived in congregate housing with other people who experienced disabilities. Although this research focus on the "bad news" didn't provide many strategies for fixing the problem, some researchers began to examine the lives of people who **were** employed, who **were** living in noninstitutional settings, and who **were** making community connections (Bogdan & Taylor, 1989; Strully & Strully, 1985). These ethnographic studies and stories about individual people pointed to one variable that seemed to be more influential than all others in predicting a "good life"—greater amounts of time spent with people without disabilities who considered the person a real friend. Not coincidentally, students who had friends without disabilities were those students who were included in regular education classes for a significant portion of their school day. Thus, although there were few research studies demonstrating the academic benefits of regular class integration, more and more families and professional organizations began to advocate for students' integration into general education classes. They believed that the most important outcome of schooling was friendships and that improved academic outcomes were a welcomed, but unanticipated benefit. (See the Preface for a review of research addressing outcomes of inclusion.) An exemplary school program might have integrated students with severe disabilities approximately 75% of the time, while the other 25% of their day was spent out of the regular class doing school jobs, receiving community-based vocational training, or returning to resource rooms for academic or other functional skills instruction. These students might have specially organized "circles of friends" (O'Brien & Forest, 1989) comprising peers who chose to support them at school and spend time with them after school.

Example of a Program Based on Integration Philosophy

Jason is a 6th grader at Maple Grove Middle School. He has severe cerebral palsy and is unable to walk, speak, or move his hands purposefully. Jason communicates through a switch-activated computer program that scans possible letters and words and allows him to make selections. Jason is transported to school on a handicapped-accessible school bus that also picks up one other student who uses a wheelchair and ten typical students from Jason's neighborhood.

Jason participates in five regular mainstream classes, receives one-on-one instruction from a resource room teacher in reading and writing, and is provided with daily physical therapy instead of participating in the regular physical education program. Jason occasionally attends evening and weekend school functions, is visited at home by classmates approximately once a month, and attends a summer camp for students with cerebral palsy. Jason's parents are fully satisfied with his program this year but are very concerned about what will happen in high school as participation in the academic curriculum becomes more dependent on prerequisite reading and writing skills.

State of the Country in the 1990s: From Integration to Inclusion

Although the struggle for integration was far from over by 1990, many families and schools were satisfied with the progress that had been made in including students with severe disabilities part-time in regular classes. They felt that partial integration provided the "best of both worlds"—the opportunity to develop and sustain friendships with typical students and a continued emphasis on job preparation that they felt was best accomplished through early and intense vocational preparation in community settings (Brown et al., 1989). They felt as if they had achieved the vision that they struggled with throughout the 1980s and could use the relative calm in the struggle to refine the nuts and bolts of assessment, IEP development, and program evaluation.

This was not to be, however. Approximately every 3–5 years, a change occurs, defining a new standard for best practices. A growing number of families, researchers, and teachers observed the benefits of partial integration for students and concluded that the next logical step was full inclusion. For some, this meant a total restructuring of education designed to merge special and regular education into one system of education for all (National Association of State Boards of Education, 1992; Stainback & Stainback, 1985; Stainback, Stainback, & Forest, 1989).

Three interrelated but distinct variables have influenced the development of this new educational paradigm, including (a) the powerful impact that friendships have had on students' lives and the belief that full-time regular class inclusion might enhance and expand those relationships (Forest, 1989; O'Brien & Forest, 1989; Strully & Strully, 1985), (b) the difficulties that young adults continue to have in trying to sustain friendships and community involvement after leaving the entitled supports of the public education system, and (c) corresponding initiatives in regular education which are supporting more adaptive curriculum and instruction within an atmosphere of greater respect for student diversity (Brookover et al., 1982; Pugach & Sapon-Shevin, 1987; Sizer, 1992; Thousand & Villa, 1992; West, 1990). Once again, the change in vision for students with severe disabilities precipitated a corresponding change in the notion of best practices in educational programs.

■□ DEVELOPMENT OF A NEW PARADIGM OF EDUCATION FOR ALL

This new model of education—full inclusion in a restructured school—needs to be articulated in unambiguous terms that offer practical guidance to all members of the school community, including students, families, teachers, administrators, and general community members. Table 1–1 illustrates the interrelationship between beliefs and practices associated with this new paradigm of restructured, inclusive schools.

Clearly, implementing full inclusion practices requires systematic and careful changes in all aspects of the educational system—in grading, teacher training, pedagogy, curriculum and materials, staff roles, and funding. These changes are not just changes in the business of special education, but rather a total reform of regular education so that it includes, not just accommodates, students who have been labeled disabled or somehow different from the norm. Given the global nature of these changes, new strategies to effect those changes are required. First and foremost, the impetus and leadership for change must come primarily from regular education. Although special educators, students, and families must be intimately involved in the process, the only assurance of permanence is for the change to originate within regular education. Fortunately, the timing is right because of a growing national movement towards school reform and restructuring which is being expanded in many places to include the needs of all students, including those with disabilities (National Association of State Boards of Education, 1992; Thousand & Villa, 1992).

■□ THE CURRENT REVOLUTION IN REGULAR EDUCATION

In general education, the focus for the last 10 years has been on educational reform to prepare future graduates for competitive jobs within a global economy in the next century. Despite the ongoing controversies about the validity of cross-national comparisons of student achievement and other measures of the effectiveness of a country's educational system, our nation as a whole has reached consensus that our schools are in trouble. There is an increasing disparity between student achievement in affluent and poor communities. Business and industry leaders yearn for students who can coherently read, write and speak and who are able to solve complex, unfamiliar problems through collaboration with other workers. And there's a general feeling that because "students are different," "families are different," and "teachers are different" in the 1990s, a dramatic response is necessary to solve our educational problems. From this realization the school restructuring

Table 1–1
Relationship between beliefs and practices in inclusive, restructured schools

Beliefs	Practices
All students have value and have something to offer the school.	Diversity is celebrated through different holidays, recognition of a variety of types of achievement—athletic, academic, volunteering, and so on.
All students benefit from learning together with others who have different talents and needs.	There is an emphasis on cooperative learning and helping one another.
Teaching practices must be adapted to fit the heterogeneous nature of the student body.	Teaching practices are utilized that are proven effective for diverse groups of learners; cooperative learning; reading and writing process; coaching rather than lecturing; active learning; individualized instruction is available to all students, not just those with disabilities.
Collaboration among teachers enhances the teaching and the learning environment.	The school provides time for teachers to work together and teachers utilize collaborative skills to develop curriculum, deliver instruction, and resolve problems.
Unless students have friends and feel worthwhile, they will be unprepared for learning and their education will be incomplete.	Intentional community building strategies are used such as devoting considerable time and energy to advisee-advisor relationships and developing circles of friends for students.
Separating students into groups based on characteristics that are traditionally devalued is counterproductive.	There are no separate classes for students with disabilities and homogeneous instructional grouping is utilized with care.

movement has been born. It has its foundation in concerns about the educational and posteducational performance of typical students, students who are at-risk because of their race or culture, and students with mild disabilities (Brookover et al., 1982; Gartner & Lipsky, 1987; Sizer, 1992). If students graduating from high school at the end of the twentieth century hope to be contributing members of a global community, they need to be able to understand and synthesize information and work collaboratively with others to identify and solve problems. For schools to adequately provide students with that knowledge and those skills, more than a cosmetic curricular facelift is needed. A total reexamination of desired student outcomes must be accompanied by a critical look at the structure of schools. This educational restructuring, whether it is called "effective schooling," "essential schooling," or simply educational reform, has been characterized by a number of ideas and principles including, but not limited to (a) curriculum driven by a small set of desired student outcomes, (b) teacher empowerment, (c) site-based management, (d) active involvement of students in the learning process, (e) increased reliance on collaboration among staff, (f) use of coaching as the dominant pedagogy, (g) use of nontraditional evaluation processes, and (h) individualization in teaching methods based on students' learning styles and needs (Pugach & Sapon-Shevin, 1987; Sizer, 1992; Thousand & Villa, 1992; West, 1990).

■□ MERGING REGULAR AND SPECIAL EDUCATION

These regular education reform and restructuring principles are also effective principles in special education. Have regular education and special education—especially as exemplified in the inclusion movement—evolved along similar paths and might they now be poised to join forces to improve educational outcomes for all students?

The U.S. Department of Education is currently funding long-term financial and training assistance to schools that are committed to the principles of school restructuring and inclusion (Nisbet & Jorgensen, 1992). Research in these experimental schools will undoubtedly generate a new set of best practices valid for all students that can provide guidance for practitioners in reformed and reforming schools. But, for now, what guidelines can practitioners follow regardless of their own school's progress on school reform or inclusion? What portions of special education practice are still valid and will contribute to a student's inclusion and preparation for adult life? Authors of national best practice documents have revised their original tools to reflect the need for guidelines that merge the best of special education reform and the best of regular education restructuring. Meyer, Eichinger and Downing (1992) revised the PQI instrument to reflect a greater commitment to full inclusion. For example, the original checklist contained the following indicator: "Students participate in heterogeneously grouped instruction, with nonhandicapped peers, at least 3 times a week." On the new checklist, item #31 states "Removal from the assigned regular classroom is considered only as a temporary measure either when absolutely necessary for health/safety reasons or because of seriously disruptive behavior that is interfering with the learning of others." Similarly, the revised version of the Vermont Best Practice Guidelines contains language that is appropriate for all students, not just those with educational handicaps (Vermont Department of Education, 1991).

■ RESPONSE TO THE REGULAR EDUCATION AND INCLUSION INITIATIVES FROM COMMUNICATION SPECIALISTS

Mirenda and Calculator (1993) advocated the regular classroom as the "point of departure" from which all decisions related to the educational placement of students with severe disabilities should commence. In attempting to meet students' individual needs through personalized curricula, these investigators noted that such attempts often remove students from the very people and settings in which targeted skills have been identified as priorities. Also lost are the opportunities for interaction and modeling intrinsic to regular classrooms.

Mirenda and Calculator's review of best practices in the provision of augmentative alternative communication (AAC) services to students with severe disabilities in regular classrooms summarized results of an earlier survey by Calculator that was completed by "experts" in education, AAC, and various related services. Survey results are summarized below. (Note: best practices relative to communication assessment and intervention are also discussed at length in Chapters 4 and 5 of this book.)

Respondents to Calculator's survey (in Mirenda & Calculator, 1993) strongly agreed that communication goals should be based on and monitored by an assessment of each individual child's abilities to meet daily communication demands. Methods of communication were viewed as effective by the extent that students' participation was enhanced in the classroom and elsewhere. This required examinations of the effect of communication systems on the number and quality of individuals' interactions with peers and adults.

Respondents agreed that communication programs should not only prepare students to participate in classrooms, but should also work toward creating environments in which such interactions are frequent and valued by all. Consistent with tenets of inclusive education, this can also include opportunities for nondisabled students to use AAC symbols and techniques in their everyday interactions (Romski & Sevcik, 1992, 1993).

It should be obvious at this point that best practices call for the incorporation of communication into existing opportunities for interaction and learning. Respondents to the survey rejected the notion that communication needs should be addressed in the form of discrete blocks, or units of time. Instead, they indicated a preference for infusing communication instruction throughout the day, basing content on the broader activities (e.g., reading, writing, art, music, and so forth) in which communication needs and opportunities arise. Similarly, they felt that communication instruction (and providing environments in which communication is present and valued) is a responsibility shared by the entire school community, and not the sole province of the SLP.

Finally, respondents' visions of best practices in AAC were consistent with procedures and philosophies associated with educational restructuring and effective schooling, discussed earlier. AAC resources were deemed best utilized when available to all students and staff.

Although students with severe disabilities certainly present special challenges in regular classrooms, their educational and related needs can best be met by teachers and others who employ instructional techniques and procedures that reflect the tremendous diversity among all students. This may require adapting the classroom environment (e.g., rearranging desks and other furniture, making appropriate work surfaces available to all students, having various forms of technology available and accessible). It may also be represented in attempts to assist students to become more active learners. For example, the extent to which students may participate in class will depend greatly on the appropriateness of fit between the students' methods of communication and those techniques called for in different classroom activities.

Students must not only be provided with methods of communication—they, their teachers, and classmates must also be encouraged to modify the curriculum (including their own individual styles and methods of interaction) to promote full participation by all students. For example, as her classmates read a story about a child who had, "A Very Bad Day," Tammy related a series of incidents to a classmate that she felt would constitute a very bad day for her. The classmate and Tammy drew pictures to represent each of Tammy's ideas. Later, the class discussed how the experiences they read about paralleled their own lives. Tammy, with cues provided by her pictures, participated in this discussion.

Finally, if students with severe disabilities are to be educated effectively in inclusive classrooms, it is critical that they develop communication skills necessary to meet classroom demands, rather than expecting all instruction to be modified to their specific learning style. Mirenda and Calculator (1993) provide suggestions for accomplishing this goal. For example, aides, classmates and others can preview assignments to predict phrases that may be useful for a student in upcoming tasks. This content can then be programmed on the student's communication aid, in the form of phrases. Phrases are expected to provide the student with more rapid responses than that afforded by constructing messages one symbol at a time.

■□ TRANSLATING BEST PRACTICES INTO PROGRAM REALITIES

What are the implications for this educational evolution for families and teachers of students with severe disabilities? How can checklists and position papers be translated into practical guidelines for making difficult decisions about placement, educational priorities, teaching strategies and allocation of support resources? A first step in this process is for professionals to sharpen their program evaluation skills so that they can assess how closely their current practices align with current best practices. The following scenarios present examples of programs that have been discussed in this chapter. As you read each one, ask yourself the following questions: (a) Do these practices demonstrate a belief in the gifts and talents of all students? (b) Do these practices promote both the social and academic inclusion of students with severe disabilities now and in the future? (c) Do these practices reflect the highest expectations for students with severe disabilities? (d) Do these practices exemplify current best practices relative to curricular design and instruction?

■□ THREE SCENARIOS

Amy's Day

Amy is a 6th grader at Hilltop Middle School. She has Rett's syndrome, which leaves her unable to speak and causes her to have a very unsteady gait, seizures, and episodes of frequent hand-wringing. One of the only purposeful movements she can make with her hands is to reach for something to eat or drink. She rides to school on a regular school bus and walks into class with her girlfriends. After a brief homeroom period, the class goes to science, but Amy picks up attendance sheets with the support of a teaching assistant. At each doorway, the teacher pauses in his or her lesson to say good morning to Amy and to hand her the attendance sheet. With hand-over-hand assistance, Amy puts each sheet into the pocket of a big apron that she wears during this activity. Amy then joins the science class about 20 minutes late. She sits with her cooperative learning group and they assist her in participating in all aspects of the class. They open her book, help her follow along with her finger, and give her hand-over-hand assistance during experiments.

After science Amy goes to social studies and participates by: (a) using eye gaze to make choices about where to sit or to select a picture representing a research topic she'd like to work on; (b) manipulating concrete materials with hand-over-hand assistance to make something that is related to the subject being studied, such as building a sugar-cube pyramid as other students are writing about Egyptian culture in their notebooks; and (c) "being part of the group" by laughing with her classmates, or going to the front of the room and holding a poster of a group project.

After a short morning recess, her classmates go to math while Amy goes to the OT's room to have a snack, brush her teeth, and swing in a vestibular stimulation net while the teaching assistant takes a break. Amy rejoins her class for French, lunch, physical education, and part of English class. During the last half hour of the day Amy receives music therapy.

Amy and one other girl are the only students with severe disabilities in this school who are included in regular classes. Other students with disabilities attend programs outside of the district or in substantially separate classes within the building. While Amy's classroom teachers do participate in curriculum planning meetings, the responsibility for coordinating Amy's education rests with the district's inclusion facilitator.

Amy attends all school functions with friends, has sleep-overs and a wide circle of support. Amy's parents are fully satisfied with her program this year but are very concerned about what will happen in junior high school and high school, as classes will be more academic, with teachers relying more on lecture than on hands-on learning.

Jordan's Day

Jordan is a lively, happy, friendly 11-year-old boy who has severe multiple disabilities. He has lived in a pediatric nursing home since he was 3, when his parents decided they could no longer care for him at home.

At 7 every morning he travels 45 minutes to an elementary school several towns away to attend the "developmental skills program." Seven other children between the ages of 3 and 15, each assigned a paraprofessional, also attend the program. A special education teacher coordinates the program and the children are visited by various itinerant specialists throughout the week, such as a physical therapist, speech-language pathologist, and an occupational therapist.

The day is organized around the seemingly endless personal care routines of the students. On arrival Jordan is fed breakfast and his teeth are brushed. Jordan has one or more therapy sessions each day. The physical therapist performs range-of-motion and neurodevelopmental techniques with him on a mat in the center of the classroom. The occupational therapist employs a large net suspended from the ceiling to conduct sensory integration activities and the speech-language pathologist conducts oral-motor stimulation activities with him. When Jordan is not engaged in therapy, personal care, or some activity of daily living, he lies on the floor or sits in a prone stander looking at or playing with pre-school toys that have been placed within his reach. Preparation for lunch, feeding, and clean up occurs between 10:30 a.m. and noon. From noon until 1 p.m. Jordan takes a nap.

In the afternoon, Jordan is taken on a walk in his stroller around the school building or out onto the school grounds. If there is a special activity going on in the school such as an assembly or holiday party, he (with all the other students in his class) joins a nearby first grade classroom. At 2:30 the van picks up Jordan and drives him back to the nursing home.

Alex's Day

Alex is a 16-year-old young man who is a 10th grader at a local high school. Shortly after Alex was born in Egypt, he had surgery to correct a minor birth defect on his scalp. There were complications (his medical records are incomplete) that resulted in a life-threatening infection. Although he recovered, he has significant hearing loss in one ear, his ability to talk is severely impaired, and he has significant learning difficulties. From the time he came to the United States (age 5) until age 15, Alex was enrolled in self-contained special education classes for students with moderate to severe disabilities. There were some early attempts to teach him to talk and read, but his records indicated that he has moderate to severe mental retardation. Last fall, facilitated communication was introduced to Alex and he demonstrated an ability to read and spell. His spelling is heavily influenced by English being a second language to him. The best way to describe his spelling is that he spells in English with an Egyptian accent! He apparently can't hear certain sounds and therefore doesn't use those sounds in spelling.

This year Alex is fully included in a regular ninth grade course of studies—English, social studies, math, science, marketing, and physical education. He uses a laptop computer to do his school work and carries a printed letter board for informal communication. He types independently most of the time but benefits from light support under his forearm when talking about subjects that make him uncomfortable.

The expectations regarding what Alex should learn in his classes are tailored to his strengths and needs. He has shown a remarkable talent for math, especially when it involves calculations and concepts grounded in repeatable patterns. In English he listens to "books on tape," other students prepare summaries of chapters and books for him, and a teaching assistant reads to him. In social studies, he is expected to learn one or two major concepts in each unit and to participate in group projects. In science, he is able to use his keen observation skills to participate in experiments. Although other students are expected to understand the chemistry of ozone depletion, Alex is expected to understand that the Earth is a planet in space. Alex enjoys his marketing class because each student works in the school store and that's where Alex is able to see his wide circle of friends every day. He helped manage the football team during the fall and goes to basketball games with friends on the weekend. Alex has indicated that he wants to work at a local car wash in the summer to earn some spending money. School staff will consult with the car wash owner and workers regarding the support that Alex might need on his first job.

■ EVALUATING PROGRAMS BASED ON BEST PRACTICE GUIDELINES

Amy's Program

Amy's program is an example of integration with some remaining vestiges of developmental and functional practices. Amy's school still operates special education programs for other students with disabilities, although Amy is included in many classroom activities and lessons. However, Amy's schedule and program have some significant differences that those of her typical classmates. The responsibility for Amy's education rests primarily with her parents, the inclusion facilitator and the paraprofessional who accompanies Amy everywhere she goes. If the same philosophy and practices continue when Amy gets to high school we can expect the amount of time that she spends in regular classes to decrease. There is no systemic restructuring of curriculum and instruction to reflect the diversity of students in the school. As soon as the curriculum becomes more "academic" at the secondary level, Amy's team are likely to look for opportunities for her to practice functional skills outside of the school building. Unless specific attention is given to facilitating Amy's relationship with her peers, the social contact between Amy and typical students will decrease. By the time she graduates from high school Amy will have moved further and further away from the mainstream and is in danger of experiencing loneliness and segregation as an adult.

Jordan's Program

Jordan's program is an example of a classroom that still clings to a developmental model, despite the evidence that the students in the program are unlikely to "make up" the lag between their skills and those of their typical peers. Jordan's whole life is characterized by relationships with professionals—by people who are paid to be with him, not by people who are his friends and choose to be with him. Jordan spends his day having things done to him, rather than being engaged in active learning. To other students in this school, Jordan is undoubtedly a stranger who they view with fear and uncertainty.

Alex's Program

Alex's program exemplifies beginning efforts at inclusion and school restructuring. While Alex receives more support services than many students at his high school, all of those services are dedicated to helping him be a fully participating member of 9th grade academics and social life. The curriculum of the school is designed "from the ground up" to reflect the diversity of learners in every classroom. Special education support teachers work collaboratively with core academic teachers to design lessons and units which allow every student to demonstrate what is learned through a variety of means. Alex isn't the only student who builds models or makes collages—these performance outcomes are options for every student in the school. While Alex has the best chance of making and keeping friends, there is still a need for those relationships to be supported by Alex, his family and school personnel.

In the next chapter, specific guidelines and strategies for planning individualized inclusive educational programs, like Alex's, will be presented. Topics to be addressed include development of individualized education plans (IEP), identifying opportunities for full participation and learning within the regular curriculum, and writing short-term objectives which reflect that curriculum context.

◼◻ REFERENCES

Antonak, R. (1988). A history of the provision of services to people who are mentally retarded. In S. Calculator & J. Bedrosian (Eds.), *Communication assessment and intervention for adults with mental retardation* (pp. 9–44). Austin, TX: Pro-Ed.

Baine, D., & Sobsey, R. (1983). Implementing transdisciplinary services for severely handicapped persons. *Special Education in Canada, 58*(1), 13–14.

Baumgart, D., Brown, L., Pumpian, I., Nisbet, J., Ford, A., Sweet, M., Messina, R., & Schroeder, J. (1982). Principle of partial participation and individualized adaptations in educational programs for severely handicapped students. *Journal of the Association for the Severely Handicapped, 7,* 17–27.

Biklen, D. (1990). Communication unbound: Autism and praxis. *Harvard Educational Review, 60*(3), 291–314.

Blatt, B., & Kaplan, F. (1966). *Christmas in purgatory*. Boston: Allyn and Bacon.

Bogdan, R., & Taylor, S. J. (1989). Relationships with severely disabled people: The social construction of humanness. *Social Problems, 36*(2), 135–148.

Brookover, W., Beamer, L., Efthim, H., Hathaway, L., Miller, J., & Tornatsky, L. (1982). *Creating effective schools: An in-service program for enhancing school learning climate and achievement.* Holmes Beach, FL: Learning Publications, Inc.

Brown, L., Branston, M. B., Hamre-Nietupski, S., Pumpian, I., Certo, N., & Gruenewald, L. (1979). A strategy for developing chronological age-appropriate and functional curricular content for severely handicapped adolescents and young adults. *Journal of Special Education, 13,* 81–90.

Brown, L., Long, E., Udvari-Solner, A., Schwartz, P., Van Deventer, P., Ahlgren, C., Johnson, F., Gruenewald, L., & Jorgensen, J. (1989). Should students with severe intellectual disabilities be based in regular or special education classrooms in home schools? *Journal of The Association for Persons with Severe Handicaps, 14,* 8–12.

Brown, L., Nietupski, J., & Hamre-Nietupski, S. (1976). The criterion of ultimate functioning in public school services for severely handicapped students. In M. A. Thomas (Ed.), *Hey! Don't forget about me: Education's investment in the severely, profoundly, and multiply handicapped* (pp. 2–15). Reston, VA: Council for Exceptional Children.

Campbell, P. (1987). The integrated programming team: An approach for coordinating professionals of various disciplines in programs for students with severe and multiple handicaps. *Journal of The Association for Persons wih Severe Handicaps, 12,* 107–116.

Education for All Handicapped Children Act of 1975, 20 U.S.C. § 1401.

Flynn, G., & Kowalczyk-McPhee, B. (1989) A school system in transition. In S. Stainback, W. Stainback, & M. Forest (Eds.), *Including all students in the mainstream of regular education.* Baltimore: Brookes Publishing Co.

Ford, A., Johnson, F., Pumpian, I., Stengert, J., & Wheeler, J. (1980). *A longitudinal listing of chronological age-apprpriate and functional activities for school aged moderately and severely handicapped students.* Madison, WI: Madison Metropolital School District.

Forest, M. (1989). *It's about relationships.* Toronto: Frontier College Press.

Gartner, A., & Lipsky, D. (1989). Beyond special education: Toward a quality system for all students. *Harvard Educational Review, 57,* 367–395.

Giangreco, M. (1986). Effects of integrated therapy: A pilot study. *Journal of The Association for Persons with Severe Handicaps, 11,* 205–208.

Gold, M. (1980). *Try another way training manual.* Champaign, IL: Research Press.

Lyon, S., & Lyon, G. (1980). Team functioning and staff development: A role release approach to providing integrated educational services for severely handicapped students. *Journal of The Association for the Severely Handicapped, 5,* 250–263.

McCormick, L., & Goldman, R. (1979). The transdisciplinary model: Implications for service delivery and personnel preparation for the severely and profoundly handicapped. *AAESPH Review, 4,* 152–161.

Meyer, L. (1987). *Program quality indicators (PQI): A checklist of most promising practices in educational programs for students with severe disabilities.* Syracuse, NY: Division of Special Education and Rehabilitation, Syracuse University.

Meyer, L., Eichinger, J., & Downing, J. (1992). *Program quaity indicators (PQI): A checklist of most promising practices in educational programs for students with severe disabilities.* Syracuse, NY: School of Education, Syracuse University.

Mirenda, P., & Calculator, S. (1993). Enhancing curricula design. *Clinics in Communication Disorders, 3,* 43–58.

Nietupski, J., Schultz, G., & Ockwood, L. (1981). The delivery of communication therapy services to severely handicapped students: A plan for change. *Journal of Association for the Severely Handicapped, 59*(1), 13–23.

Nisbet, J., & Jorgensen, C. (1992). *Including students with disabilities in systemic efforts to restructure schools.* U.S. Department of Education, Office of Special Education and Rehabilitative Services. Grant # H023R20018.

O'Brien, J., & Forest, M. (1989). *Action for inclusion.* Toronto, Ontario: Centre for Integrated Education, Frontier College.

PARC v. Commonwealth of PA, 334 F. Supp. 1257 (E.D. Penn, 1971).

Pugach, M., & Sapon-Shevin, M. (1987). New agendas for special education policy: What the national reports haven't said. *Exceptional Children, 53,* 295–299.

Romski, M., & Sevcik, R. (1992). Developing augmented language in children with severe mental retardation. In S. Warren & J. Reichle (Eds.), *Causes and effects in communication intervention.* Baltimore: Paul H. Brookes.

Romski, M., & Sevcik, R. (1993). Language through augmented means. In A. Kaiser & D. Gray (Eds.), *Enhancing children's communication: Research foundations for intervention.* Baltimore: Paul H. Brookes.

Sailor, W., Gee, K., Goetz, L., & Graham, N. (1988). Progress in educating students with the most severe disabilities: Is there any? *Journal of The Association for Persons with Severe Handicaps, 13,* 87–99.

Sears, C. (1981). The transdisciplinary approach: A process for compliance with Public Law 94-142. *Journal of the Association for the Severely Handicapped, 6,* 22–29.

Sizer, T. (1992). *Horace's school: Redesigning the American high school.* Boston: Houghton Mifflin Co.

Stainback, S., Stainback, W., & Forest, M. (Eds.). (1989). *Educating all students in the mainstream of regular education.* Baltimore: Paul Brookes Publishing Co.

Stainback, W., & Stainback, S. (1984). A rationale for the merger of special and regular education. *Exceptional Children, 51,* 102–111.

Strully, J., & Strully, C. (1985). Friendship and our children. *Journal of The Association for Persons with Severe Handicaps, 10,* 224–227.

Thousand, J. (1987). *Best practice guidelines for students with intensive educational needs.* Burlington: University of Vermont Center for Developmental Disabilities.

Thousand, J., & Villa, R. (1992). *Restructuring for caring and effective education.* Baltimore: Brookes Publishing Co.

Vermont Department of Education. (1991). *Best practice guidelines for meeting the needs of all students in local schools.* Burlington, VT: Instructional Support Service Unit, State Department of Education.

West, F. (1990). Educational collaboration in the restructuring of schools. *Journal of Educational and Psychological Consultation, 1*(1), 23-40.

Wolfensberger, W. (1972). *The principle of normalisation in human services.* Toronto: National Institute on Mental Retardation.

Yoder, D., & Calculator, S. (1981). Some perspectives on intervention stategies for persons with developmental disorders. *Journal of Autism and Developmental disorders, 11,* 107–123.

Developing Individualized Inclusive Educational Programs

Cheryl M. Jorgensen

■□ INTRODUCTION

Traditional texts dealing with communication programming describe comprehensive strategies for conducting communication assessments, developing communication programs, and evaluating the impact of communication services. Some guidelines are generally given to speech-language pathologists (SLPs) for how those assessments, programs, and evaluation strategies can be integrated into a student's overall program. This practice, common to many related service disciplines, has resulted in fragmentation of students' programs. Related service goals and objectives oftentimes "drive" a student's whole educational program. Classroom teachers look at an individualized education program (IEP) outline and see communication goals, fine motor goals, large motor goals, personal care goals, and so forth. Can we fault them for exclaiming "Switch activation? Toileting? Object permanence? Stair climbing? I teach social studies in this class. This student doesn't belong here!"

In the middle chapters of this book we argue for a different program design strategy—one that reflects the values and best practices outlined in the Prologue, Preface, and first chapter. That is, although communication is an essential component of a quality life for everyone (including students with severe disabilities), it cannot be considered or even adequately addressed outside of a broader focus and commitment to students' educational programs which reflect inclusion into regular, age-appropriate classrooms. From a practical standpoint, this means that assessing students' communication repertoires should occur within a broader assessment of students' overall functioning in integrated settings. It means that "communication programming" per se, must involve a set of teaching strategies and other supports employed to assist students in benefitting from the regular education curriculum and other school and community activities. And it means that valid assessment of student learning and program quality views success in communication as inextricably tied to success in school.

This chapter presents (a) new ways of getting to know students with severe disabilities which emphasizes their gifts not their disabilities, (b) a process for identifying the focus of a student's education for a current school year, (c) examples of short-term objectives that reflect learning and participating in typical classrooms and environments, (d) a format for brainstorming classroom participation options, and (e) strategies for forming peer supports and encouraging friendships.

■□ WHY IT'S IMPORTANT TO GET TO KNOW STUDENTS IN NEW WAYS: AN EXAMPLE FROM SOUHEGAN COOPERATIVE SCHOOL DISTRICT

On September 1, 1992, after 16 years of attending segregated special education programs, Brad and five classmates with severe disabilities arrived at Souhegan High School to begin their first school year in regular classes.[1] Imagine that as the district's SLP, the rest of the special education team is looking to you for guidance regarding the development of Brad's "communication program." Where would you start? Might his cumulative folder and other past records provide some clue as to how Brad communicates, what methods have been successful in the past, and what the focus of this year's program ought to be? If you browsed through his voluminous records, you would learn that Brad was born prematurely in 1976 and that his parents were told that something was "wrong" shortly after his birth. His facial features were dysmorphic, he had microcephaly, and was given oxygen at birth. He never learned to talk and all of his developmental milestones were significantly delayed or never reached. Brad received no formal early intervention as an infant or toddler, but at the age of 3 he was enrolled in a self-contained preschool program administered by The Easter Seals Society. Although the class Brad was in focused on teaching students the usual developmental skills appropriate for typically developing preschoolers—colors, counting, play and social skills, dressing, eating—Brad's significantly challenging behavior often interfered with his participation in the group and he spent a great deal of time being "behavior modified." Until he was 12, his elementary school experience was in a class for students labeled trainably mentally retarded. At that time, he moved into a self-contained class at a public middle school in which his program concentrated on such functional skills as cooking, cleaning, shopping, and so forth. During the course of his schooling, Brad was introduced to many different communication systems including AmerInd, American Sign Language (ASL), natural gestures, and picture communication boards. Intellectual and communication testing was limited to informal observations and other procedures, as well as administration of adaptive behavior scales because of his "refusal to cooperate with the tester" in more formal assessment situations. The communication goals on the most recent IEP included (a) improve ability to make choices, (b) express frustration in a socially acceptable manner, (c) learn 10 new signs relating to community safety awareness, and (d) combine two signs to

---

[1] The new public school is a member of the Coalition of Essential Schools, founded by Theodore Sizer (1992). It subscribes to a philosophy of full inclusion. There are no rooms or programs solely for students with disabilities; there is limited tracking (in math and some advanced placement courses); and students are grouped heterogeneously in most other classes.

request objects or attention. The only signs that Brad initiates are for eat, coffee, bathroom, and music.

Based on this information, do you know what Brad will need in the way of communication programming to enable him to participate in 9th grade social studies? To join an after-school club? To have a conference with his guidance counselor and choose his classes for the second semester? To hang out with his fellow 9th graders during free periods? Are you worried about what others will expect you to be able to provide relative to a means for Brad to communicate?

When students are included in regular classes or when teams are planning to move a student from a segregated to an integrated class, "what's important to know about a student" takes on a whole new meaning. In Brad's case, his team (including the regular class teachers from four core subject areas) generated a list of questions that reflected their view of "what's important to know." They included:

1. Can he use the bathroom independently?
2. Is he in any danger of hurting himself or others?
3. How does he tell people he needs or wants something?
4. What is his personality like? Calm, excitable, interested, irritable, cooperative?
5. Can he get around the school independently?
6. How will he get to school?
7. Can he read? What can we assume that he knows about 9th grade subject areas?
8. Does he dress appropriately?
9. How do we communicate with Brad?
10. How much do we tell the other students about Brad's past or current situation?
11. Does Brad understand what we say to him? Do we have to speak to him differently than other students?
12. How will he do his school work, if he doesn't write?

Would you find the answers to these questions in Brad's file? From the results of a standardized test? From a short observation of Brad the first few days of school?

The answer is, obviously, no. This team needs new ways to learn about Brad as a person, new ways to figure out what he knows and can do now, new values to guide their decisions about what's important for him to learn as a 9th grader, and new strategies for working together to help him achieve those goals. The most important first step for the team is to begin to see Brad in a new light, to begin a process of telling "new Brad stories," which will promote, not hinder, everyone's view of him as a student who is able to be successfully included in this school.

The strategies that follow are appropriate to use when: (a) students are currently in segregated settings and teams are planning for their inclusion into a regular class; (b) students are included part-time in a regular class and teams feel a need to "start-over" with their understanding of the student; or (c) a student is already included, but it makes sense to think about the student in a new light, such as when the student is making an important transition to a new setting where he or she isn't known by many teachers or students.

■□ TELLING NEW STORIES AND THE SEARCH FOR CAPACITY

There are no ready-made "assessment tools" for getting to know students and identifying what they need to benefit from inclusion in regular education classes. There are, however, some processes for asking new questions, and three of the most widely known are discussed here.

M.A.P.S.

Marsha Forest and Judith Snow (Vandercook, York, & Forest, 1989) pioneered a process—M.A.P.S.—for linking these conversations about the past with a discussion of an individual's desirable future. Conducting a M.A.P.S. session with a student, family, and friends is a focused way of discovering their thoughts about the student and a new school situation. The student and family members are asked the following questions:

1. Who is this person? (Described in "regular" words, not special education language)
2. What is this individual's history?
3. What is his or her dream?
4. What is the nightmare, if the dream doesn't come true?
5. What are the person's gifts?
6. What does the person need right now (this year) to have a good life?

7. What needs to be done by us (student, parents, teachers, peers, other support staff) to help the person realize those needs?

Information from the M.A.P.S. session, supplemented with observations (in school, in the community, and at home) and evaluations, can then be utilized to make decisions about support needs, adaptive technology, training for staff, and student involvement in extracurricular activities, as well as to target specific learning objectives for the current school year.

The following example illustrates the information that one team obtained from using the M.A.P.S. process with a student, Joshua. Josh is a 10-year-old boy who is currently included in a 5th grade class. The team learned the following information about Josh from conducting a M.A.P.S. session in the spring before Josh's transition to his neighborhood school that fall. Josh, his mother and sisters, his current and former teachers, and selected 5th grade classmates answered the following questions:

1. Who is Josh? He has great rhythm; uses facial expression to communicate his wants, needs, and feelings; is happy; becomes bored when not doing something interesting; is affectionate; is in great health; is patient; needs much help with personal hygiene and other activities of daily living; is fun-loving; is handsome and cute; moves around by walking; and doesn't appear to know letters, how to read, or do math.

2. What is his history? He had a normal birth; developmental disabilities diagnosed at 6 months; attended early intervention and special education preschool programs; attended out-of-district, self-contained special education programs from the ages of 5–8; was partially included in regular class in out-of-district 4th grade and is fully included in regular class in neighborhood 5th grade; parents are divorced and Josh lives with his mom and has two older sisters who are in college.

3. What is his and his mother's dream? His mom said that her main priority is that Josh have real friendships. She also identified as important having a place to live with people he likes that is not an institution or his family's home; having a paying job in a real work setting; being able to move around the community, enjoy the outdoors, attend musical events; being safe and secure; and being respected and liked by people in the community.

4. What is the nightmare? Josh's mom easily identified having to leave his home and reside in a group home if she becomes burned out or living in an institution or a group home as the nightmare. Additionally, she hoped he wouldn't be abused or be lonely.

5. What are his gifts? People are drawn to him; he can bring kids together who normally don't get along; he is friendly; he likes to try new activities; he loves books; he is easygoing and adjusts to new situations pretty well; and he has a mom who is a strong advocate for him.

6. What does he need to be successfully included? Josh needs a teacher who likes him and treats him normally; a communication system that helps people know more about what Josh is thinking, wanting, feeling; a full-time teaching assistant to help out in his classes; friends to spend time with in and outside of school; access to community activities; more respite for mom (e.g. time away from mom on the weekends).

7. What do team members need to do to facilitate achievement of his dream and to successfully include him in 5th grade this year? Principal, mom, and teacher need to work together to recruit and hire a teaching assistant who understands how to facilitate Josh's inclusion; principal needs to find substitutes so that team members can attend training workshops; 5th grade teacher will contact members of his church to see if there are any high school boys who would be Josh's companion and help him get involved in recreation department activities on the weekend; integration facilitator (support teacher) will talk to students and organize a "circle of friends" for Josh; and SLP will spend 2 half-days with Josh in school and 2 hours after school with him as a first step in developing a communication system for him.

Personal Futures Planning

Beth Mount developed a process for planning students' educational programs and after-school plans called Personal Futures Planning (Mount, 1987). The process begins by simply talking with students and their families about their past—their own unique history. Professionals often find out that early experiences in the traditional institutions of medicine and education have robbed families and individuals with disabilities of the same kinds of hopes and dreams that other parents have. When their child is born, parents of students with severe disabilities are often told to abandon their thoughts of the future ("Your child may not live past infancy") or to severely curtail their expectations ("Children like this rarely are able to live on their own once they grow up").

Listening to families talk about the past is an important way for every staff member to establish rapport. It's essential that staff acknowledge families' experiences as unique and valid and that they resist the temptation to excuse the predictions of experts by saying "Well, we didn't know better at the time." Simply listening to families and acknowledging their feelings is essential. After staff learn about students' and families' past experiences, they then facilitate the development of a well-rounded description of the student's interests, talents, social relationships, current activities, and so forth. Like the M.A.P.S. process, students and families are then given permission to speak about the dreams they never thought were possible. Examples of dream statements that are common to many students and families are: "I want my daughter to live here at home with us if we can get enough help." "I want to learn to drive a car." "I want to have friends." "I want to go to college." "I want to earn my own money."

Unlike M.A.P.S., which usually is accomplished in one or two meetings, Personal Futures Planning usually occurs over a long period of time with the student or adult with a disability together with the individual's support network of family, friends and support staff.

C.O.A.C.H.

Another systematic planning process for getting to know students is incorporated into the C.O.A.C.H. model (Giangrego, Iverson, & Cloninger, 1993).[2] C.O.A.C.H. is a family-focused team process which results in: (a) a set of discipline-free annual goals; (b) measureable short-term objectives which support those goals; (c) a list of supports the student will need in order to reach those goals within an inclusive regular classroom; and (d) preliminary plans for how the student will participate within the regular education curriculum. The C.O.A.C.H. process begins with a student/

---

[2] When it was first developed, C.O.A.C.H. stood for Cayuga-Onondaga Assessment for Children with Handicaps. In its most recent edition the acronym was changed to Choosing Options and Accommodations for Children with Handicaps.

family interview in which several quality-of-life indicators are explored, including, among others, the student's current living situation, health status and well-being, and how and with whom the student spends free time. The student and family are encouraged to decide which indicators should be a priority for improvement during a current school year and then to select program goals and objectives based on those values.

When staff members have a more complete picture of the student's likes and dislikes, interests, personality quirks, and so forth, it's important to incorporate this new information into formal and informal conversations with other school staff and students. Consider Brad's case as an example of the need to view students in a positive light during planning for inclusion into a regular class. Before I (CJ) had even met Brad, someone approached me in the hallways and warned me that "Brad is a biter—he got me last week. Have you been bitten yet?" To counteract the effect of comments like these, some teams decide to start every meeting with a "good story" that celebrates an accomplishment of a student. They make sure to speak of students with disabilities as having the personalities distinct from the characteristics of their disability. Speaking directly with the person who makes disparaging comments about students may make them aware of the effect that their language has on other students' or teachers' perception of the student with the disability. Adhering to "people first" language involves using disability-related descriptors as modifiers as in "students with autism" or "the student who uses a wheelchair." Because teachers and other staff members are accustomed to referring to students by well-known characteristics (Marissa is the superintendent's daughter; John is the punter on the football team; Karen is the girl who did the caricatures in the faculty lounge), teachers need a shorthand way to refer to students with disabilities as well. In Brad's case it should be, "you know Brad, he's the kid whose stepfather drives the school bus", instead of "you know Brad, he's the one who bites his aide." It's a process of rehumanizing people who none of us have known because they were out-of-sight and out-of-mind for years.

■□ THE PROGRAM DEVELOPMENT PROCESS

Getting to know students through M.A.P.S. sessions or by using Personal Futures Planning can be done any time—not just as a preliminary step to developing a student's IEP. Strategies for relating IEPs to broader planning efforts and quality of life issues are complex and vary according to state and local policies. Suggestions for doing so are provided in the sections to follow.

The process of getting to know students in a new light can be implemented at any time during a school year, with a student who is currently in an integrated or segregated school setting. Table 2–1 describes the entire program development process, which reflects best practices (as summarized in Chapter 1) and the authors' experiences working with New Hampshire schools since 1985. The

TABLE 2-1
Program development process

Step 1. Describe the student's capacity and needs by using M.A.P.S., talking with the student, peers, teachers, and family members.

Step 2. Identify anticipated barriers to the student's inclusion and develop plans and timelines to address those barriers (training for teachers, initial projections regarding hiring or reassignment of support staff, meeting with transportation company).

Step 3. Develop a process for facilitating friendships and peer supports.

Step 4. Choose priority learning goals for current school year.

Step 5. Specify how the student will participate within the regular class, other school and extracurricular activities, and revise need for support.

Step 6. Develop short-term objectives based on observation of the student's current skills, a discrepancy analysis of the skills required to participate in class and social situations, and other in-depth assessment information.[a]

Step 7. Develop teaching and curriculum modification strategies based on student's learning style and the teaching style(s) of the regular class teacher(s). This step is ongoing and needs to be continually revised based on what is being taught in the regular classroom.[b]

Step 8. Evaluate the student's inclusion and the effectiveness of instruction in helping the student achieve his priority learning outcomes.

[a] See Chapter 4 for a description of assessmment procedures associated with communication issues and inclusion.

[b] See Chapter 5 for instructional procedures for linking communication to successful inclusion.

most important concepts associated with the process are (a) to inform and involve the student and family members throughout the process, (b) to adhere as closely as possible to the regular education process and timetable for class assignments and student planning, and (c) to strive for balance between program breadth (participation) and depth (specific learning objectives).

Timing

The chronology of events surrounding the development of a student's individualized educational program and priority learning objectives (IEP) is determined by the practices and regulations of the district and state in which the student resides as well as by the student's current and projected placement. Some districts develop students' IEPs in the spring in preparation for promotion to the next grade. Others use students' birthdates as stepping-off points for annual evaluation and IEP development activities. As the expectation for regular class inclusion becomes more commonplace, program planning for students with disabilities ought to more nearly parallel planning activities for typical students. In the spring, elementary teachers usually meet as grade-level teams to discuss student needs and make a recommendation to the principal for class assignments for the following year. At the middle and high school levels, students without disabilities work together with their parents and guidance counselors to select courses based on requirements for graduation and postschool work or educational plans. Generalized planning for students with disabilities should be initiated at the same time, yielding (a) information required by the next year's teachers and team members to plan the supports and services that the student will need; (b) identification of training needs of school staff that should be addressed before the beginning of the school year; and (c) plans for conducting in-class and in-school observations in the fall from which specific goals, objectives, and teaching strategies can then be developed, implemented, evaluated, and revised on an ongoing basis.

This next section briefly describes the steps in the program development process, primarily through examples of students who have been successfully included in New Hampshire schools. (The first step in the process, getting to know the student, has been described at length in previous sections of this chapter.)

Step 2: Identify Barriers to Inclusion

Even before a student is included, team members should anticipate barriers to the student's successful inclusion. This brainstorming can occur during the spring (or whenever inclusion planning
is begun) and may lead to other planning activities. Selected team
members should meet the student and parents and do both a
school (current placement) and home visit. Discussion with
the student's current team ought to include questions about the
student's personality, likes and dislikes, any important medical or
health issues, and their recommendations regarding the grade, and
if relevant, teacher, for the student. Some strategies for approaching the neighborhood school principal and for introducing the student to prospective classmates have been described by others
(Forest & O'Brien, 1990; Schaffner & Buswell, 1991; Tashie, Jorgensen
& Schuh, 1993).

These preliminary discussions often lead to other related planning and preparatory activities such as: (a) training workshops for
teachers (on topics such as curriculum modification, augmentative
and alternative communication, behavior management, rationale
for inclusion); (b) student-specific consultation from outside sources
(e.g., to develop specialized AAC systems or behavior management
plans); (c) acquisition of materials and/or equipment; (d) hiring of
additional support staff for the teachers who will have the student
in class; or (e) discussing and addressing policies that may seem
to inhibit the students' inclusion (e.g., prohibitions against students
with impaired mobility riding the regular school bus, prerequisite
coursework for enrollment in particular high school courses, funding that promotes more restrictive placements).

Step 3: Facilitate Friendships and Peer Support

In a 1990 report on life for individuals with disabilities in the state
of New Hampshire, the most commonly listed problem stated by
those individuals was loneliness (New Hampshire Developmental
Disabilities Council, 1989). Even though New Hampshire's adult
service system for adults with disabilities (developmental, vocational, and mental health) are nationally ranked in the top five in
the country, something is clearly missing in the lives of adults and
children with disabilities. For school-age children, parents indicate
that their children's need for friendship outweighs any of their

concerns about "programs" (B. Dixon, personal communication, November 1, 1992). Even when students were first included in regular classes in New Hampshire, teams did not focus on the student's peer relationships, unless parents pushed the issue or students looked conspicuously isolated. We now recognize the importance of focusing on friendships and peer support from the beginning of the inclusion process. Strully and Strully (1989) state:

> Friendships are indeed at the heart of what we all need for one another. It is our friendships that enable us to be active and protected community members. Friendships help ensure that being a part of the community, rather than just being in the community, is a reality for everyone! (p. 68)

Why do students with disabilities need to have friendships and social relationships facilitated for them? Because most typical students are hampered by their lack of experience in having friends with disabilities (and sometimes also by their attitudes and lack of knowledge), there is a need to "intentionally facilitate community" between typical students and students with disabilities (M. Forest, personal communication, May, 1989). Many people think that when students with severe disabilities are included in regular classes, friendships and other student-to-student relationships happen automatically. People are eager to dismiss strategies for facilitating and encouraging friendships because they may seem too reminiscent of the mainstreaming era (e.g. "special friends" or "peer buddies") (Perske & Perske, 1988). On the contrary, when students are fully included in regular classes, there is a compelling need to actively facilitate friendships, so that students who are physically and academically integrated do not become "islands in the mainstream"—physically present but socially isolated (Biklen, 1985, p. 189). And the connection between having friends and education? Every teacher knows that students who feel isolated and have no friends cannot possibly reach their potential as learners or as people.

There are two strategies for encouraging budding friendships and helping to assure that students have a wide range of supportive social relationships in schools and in the community.

Formal Support Circles

The process of facilitating friendship circles is not easily described and doesn't lend itself to a neat 6-step recipe. A description of how one friendship circle functioned highlights the essential values and some of the strategies that have been successful.

Jason is a 10-year-old boy in the 4th grade at his neighborhood school. He previously attended a self-contained, noncategorical program in another school within his home district. This is his first year of being fully included and he is experiencing a number of academic and social difficulties. Jason's experiences support the notion that not having friends and feeling isolated are detrimental to success in school.

Jason's early years were fairly uneventful, although his mother now remembers that he reached his early physical developmental milestones later than her other children. As a preschooler he went to a babysitter's house and during his school district's prekindergarten screening, he was found to be several years behind his age peers in language development and motor abilities. After kindergarten, he was tested by the district's multidisciplinary evaluation team and labeled educationally handicapped with accompanying speech and language impairment. Despite three years of special education instruction in a small classroom, his reading and math skills remained at the kindergarten level. Three years ago when Jason was 8, he and his two younger brothers were diagnosed with Duchenne's Muscular Dystrophy. Shortly after the diagnosis, Jason's parents divorced and both remarried. His parents have a very strained relationship, are struggling to cope with having three young children with muscular dystrophy, and are very economically needy after losing their jobs when the local Air Force base closed.

Jason's physical therapist predicts that although Jason walked independently in September, his motor abilities will regress significantly throughout the course of the year and he will need to use a wheelchair full-time within six months. Jason is meeting with a guidance counselor once a week to discuss his feelings about having muscular dystrophy, the possibility of an early death, his parents' divorce, and so forth, and according to Jason and his parents, he doesn't have any friends from school.

Although some people might not consider Jason to be a candidate for a circle of friends, he liked the idea of being in a club with some classmates with the goal of making some after-school and weekend connections. To that end, Jason's teacher spoke to his class one day while Jason was having physical therapy. Her presentation included the following information (student's comments have been omitted):

As all of you know, Jason B. is having a tough time this year because it's becoming more and more difficult for him to walk on his
own. Can some of you tell me how you would be feeling if you
were in Jason's shoes? Jason would like to start a club of kids who
would be willing to meet with him and some of us teachers once
a week to see if there are any ways that we could help Jason deal
with his situation. Is there anyone in this class who might like to
meet with us during recess today to discuss this?

Nine students raised their hands and after lunch that day,
Jason joined those nine classmates for a discussion facilitated by
the guidance counselor and Jason's teacher. The counselor helped
Jason express to his classmates that "I don't have any friend, I want
to make some new friends and I'm scared that I won't be able to
walk anymore." Immediately, the students began to offer conso-
lation to Jason, several of the boys came over to him, put their
arms around him and said that they'd be glad to help. The guidance counselor told the kids that they'd first have to come up with
a name for their club and that they would be meeting once a week
in school. One boy suggested the "J-team" and Jason liked it immediately. At the end of the recess period, the guidance counselor handed out permission slips for the students to participate in
a M.A.P.S. session the following week and the club was on its way.

Over the course of the next several months, Jason's team met
once a week and helped figure out a number of problematic issues such as how Jason would get his wheelchair out onto the
soccer field, who would push him so he could play soccer during
recess, and where Jason's dad could get some technical help in
building a safe sidecar for his motorcycle. Jason received several
birthday party invitations, seems happier in school, and his family feels as if they are getting help with the issues that concern
them most.

The role of the guidance counselor or any other adult who
assumes responsibility for facilitating Jason's circle is: (a) to plan
one short, fun activity for the team in case they seem to need some
help organizing themselves during their weekly meeting; (b) to
inform Jason's parents about plans the students are discussing so
that they don't get too far into a great idea without knowing if
Jason's parents will give him permission to do it; and (c) to facilitate each week's discussion of problems that Jason (or the other
students) is facing and how the kids might help solve it.

Some people may wonder why typical students would ever want to participate in this process? Is it realistic to expect them to give this kind of commitment to one of their classmates? The short answer is that "some will and some won't!" In the course of facilitating circles around the state of New Hampshire, we've discovered that people—children and adults alike—have an untapped capacity to care about the quality of life of people with disabilities, and perhaps, more importantly, that they have a keen sense of justice that is violated when people are excluded from participating in the mainstream of school and community life. During the 1991–1992 school year, a survey about inclusion was administered to more than 600 elementary age students in the Mascoma Valley School District. Analysis of the responses showed that 80% of elementary age students identified the concept of fairness (in adult terms, social justice) as a major reason why they felt their peers with disabilities ought to be in school and in regular classes alongside them (C. Burmeister, personal communication, April 1, 1992). Many schools suffer from the inability to make all kinds of kids feel a sense of belonging. Many students feel that they need to justify their sense of worth and belonging by being smart, athletic, pretty, thin, or compliant. The values supporting inclusion (unconditional acceptance) and the strategy of friendship circles speak to all students in language that they understand. Perhaps they feel that by supporting a classmate's struggle to belong, they are making their school a place where they, too, can feel good about themselves without being perfect.

Circles can be facilitated by the student with the disability, by a friend or advocate, by a professional (such as an SLP), by a member of the student's family, or by any person who is interested in becoming part of the student's life. People in the circle are willing participants, they don't get academic credit or volunteer certificates, and membership can change over the course of time. Ultimately the student with the disability is in control of his or her circle and is given the final say in its operation.

Individuals who wish to do more reading about circles are referred to resources cited in the Appendix.

Encouraging Informal Natural Supports

Although circles of friends provide more formal kinds of support, everyone has a diverse array of other supports in their lives that connect them to their community and provide practical and emotional safety nets. For most adults, these supports are spouses or lovers, parents and siblings, close friends, co-workers, and various "experts" we call upon periodically such as therapists, accountants, plumbers, physicians, and so forth.

The term "natural supports" has been coined to mean primarily nonpaid people who provide support to people with disabilities. In inclusive schools, Jorgensen (1992) expanded the definition to mean:

> those components of an educational program—philosophy, policies, people, materials and technology, and curricula—that are used to enable all students to be fully participating members of regular classroom, school, and community life. Natural supports bring [students] closer together as friends and learning partners rather than isolating them. (p. 183)

When students with disabilities become members of regular classes and regular schools it is imperative that their teachers create environments and opportunities in which students learn to support one another. In the long run, students who have been included and who have been supported primarily by peers are better prepared to deal with the demands of community life. The literature analyzing outcomes associated with supported employment, in which the supports are provided primarily by paid agency staff, illustrate that reliance on professional staff actually inhibits the development of social relationships with co-workers and other community members. In those instances where individuals with disabilities were socially integrated at the worksite and after work, support was being provided mainly by nonpaid staff (Nisbet & Hagner, 1988).

Examples of how students with disabilities can be naturally supported in school and the role of professional staff in encouraging and supporting these natural alliances are presented in Table 2–2.

Doesn't this list merely reflect the ways that students without disabilities work together and help one another every day? The process of inclusive education is simply including students with disabilities in the same classrooms, activities and life experiences as typical students and providing them with the supports necessary to enable them to derive meaning from those experiences.

When thinking about how to encourage students to provide assistance to one another, it's important to use common sense and to guard against stigmatizing the student with the disability by the

TABLE 2–2

Examples of interdependent learning and peer supports between typical students and students with severe disabilities

1. Providing partial physical assistance in the lunchroom, during science lab, home economics, industrial arts
2. Conferencing during writing time
3. Helping a student move arms and legs during physical education exercise routines
4. Interpreting communication attempts for other listeners
5. Offering reminders about good behavior
6. Studying together
7. Making instructional materials for other students
8. Reading to one another
9. Providing encouragement and physical support to a friend who uses a communication device
10. Offering a friend choices using his or her augmentative communication system
11. Playing interactive computer and board games together
12. Assigning valued roles to every member of one's cooperative learning group
13. Working together on group projects which utilize the strengths of every team member
14. Giving a friend a ride home after an after-school activity

Source: Adapted from "Natural Supports in Inclusive Schools: Curricular and Teaching Strategies" by C. Jorgensen in *Natural Supports in School, at Work, and in the Community for People with Severe Disabilities* (pp. 179–215) edited by J. Nisbet, 1992, Baltimore: Paul H. Brookes Publishing Co.. Copyright 1992 by Paul H. Brookes. Adapted by permission.

way that assistance is provided. Guidelines for achieving this balance are presented in Table 2–3.

Step 4: Choose Priority Learning Goals for Current School Year

One of the most frustrating tasks for families and team members is the identification and selection of goals to include on the student's IEP. Many schools that are successfully including students wish that they could just stop the planning process prior to this step! They are confused about how to integrate systematic instruction and evaluation—which sometimes feel like leftovers from self-contained, separate classes—with the new focus on participation,

TABLE 2–3
Guidelines for promoting interdependence within the classroom

1. Make sure that one student is not being singled out to receive assistance all the time. Make helping and cooperation an expectation for everyone in the class. A speech pathologist can say, "Does everyone in this group understand the directions? Let's go around and repeat the steps of the assignment."

2. When planning lessons in which some students will need assistance, think first of using other students to provide help before assigning an adult to the student with disabilities.

3. When the assistance of a specialist is needed, plan for how that person will work with small groups of students. The philosophy that all members of the educational team are responsible for the learning of all students should be maintained. For example, an SLP might work with a reading group on oral reading expression or on word-attack strategies. Some students could be prompted to read with expression, others could be taught strategies for decoding new words, while another student could be urged to articulate more clearly the names of the pictures in the story.

4. Be honest with students about not having all the answers and enlist their help in solving problems. The teacher might say, "We're starting our unit on the solar system next week. Today I'd like each group to come up with an idea for a learning center about the nine planets in our solar system so that everyone in our class will be able to partici-pate. We'll share our ideas in a half-hour."

5. Teach students to help one another learn. Too often teachers or therapists who are very skilled at teaching forget that their greatest gift is to teach their skills to students so that they become good literary critics of their peers' work or effective listeners for students who have communication difficulties.

friendships, and a more natural way of teaching. The following example illustrates the frustration when team members try to develop a new kind of regular-class IEP without understanding why they must adopt a new paradigm or without having a model for the new process.

Jamie's IEP

Not long ago, I was asked to provide assistance to a team struggling with the development of an IEP and regular education plan for an 8-year-old boy with Fragile X syndrome. When I arrived at the meeting location, I was met by no less than 12 team members, including the boy's mother. Six individual conversations were taking place and I saw that each team member had brought a list of goals to the meeting. The mom handed out her list of the 52 goals she wanted the team to address and each additional team member then took a turn reading at least half a dozen additional goals to the assembled group. When everyone had taken a turn, they all looked at me and the special education director asked, "We are really unsure about how to write an IEP for Jamie now that he is in 2nd grade. It would take us a week of meetings to plow through these goals and try to come to some consensus about which are most important. What should we do?"

I asked everyone to put away the goal sheets that were spread out on the table in front of them. I turned to Jamie's mom and asked, "What are the four most important things you'd like Jamie to accomplish this year?" She paused for a few seconds and answered deliberately "I'd like him to get invited to a birthday party. I'd like him to be able to write his name and address. I would like to see him use some kind of communication system reliably and I would like him to make friends." I asked Jamie's classroom teacher the same question and she quickly responded "I'd like him to be able to be in a large group of children without being disruptive. I hope that he'll learn to enjoy books and writing. And I wish that he'd initiate contact with other children without the need for an adult to be involved in the process."

There were Jamie's priority learning goals for the school year! I asked the group if anyone had any objection to these goals and if everyone thought that Jamie could reasonably achieve some mastery of each one. The group members nodded their heads and we set up a time to meet to discuss a process for writing short-term objectives based on classroom- and curriculum-based assessment of Jamie in a variety of regular class lessons and activities. The need for and role of related service input and staff would take place during these discussions, as was the original intent of P.L. 94–142 when the term "related" was chosen.

If all parents and team members were able to quickly come to consensus as this team did, the determination of priority learning goals would be a short and sweet process. Because of team members' varied perspectives and the difficulty that many people have in giving up their discipline-specific goals, use of a process such as the C.O.A.C.H., which was explained previously in this chapter (Giangreco, Cloninger, & Iverson, 1993) may facilitate this process.

In brief, the C.O.A.C.H. process gives families the ultimate control over the selection of 8 broadly stated goals for the IEP, instructs team members in a method for writing short-term objectives that support progress toward each goal, and then gives a model for determining how the student will participate in the broader regular education curriculum.

Returning to the example of 10-year-old Josh, his mother determined that the following eight broad priorities should form the basis for developing the annual goals and short-term objectives on his IEP:

1. Expanding his ability to make choices
2. Sustaining interactions with other children
3. Learning the school building and routine
4. Understanding one-to-one correspondence in everyday situations
5. Making friends
6. Managing his own belongings at school
7. Spending leisure time with friends
8. Doing a school job on a weekly basis

Although each of these priorities may reflect a learning outcome generally associated with a particular discipline (e.g. "spending leisure time with friends" from the leisure and recreation domain; "sustaining interactions" from the communication or social skills domains), they are broad enough in scope to be addressed by all professionals in many situations and settings throughout the school day. Rewriting these priorities as annual goals merely entails specifying the behavior that Josh's mom and other team members expect him to demonstrate at the end of the year, and the context(s) within which people expect him to demonstrate it. Josh's priorities written as IEP goals are:

1. Within real life situations such as choosing food in the lunchroom, selecting books in the library, or picking friends to be on his team in gym, Josh will make a choice from among five choices within each category.
2. When talking with a responsive peer, Josh will take three conversational turns using his communication book or natural gestures.
3. When doing errands, on trips to the boys' rooms, or at other times, Josh will independently walk to familiar rooms within the school building.
4. Josh will demonstrate an understanding of one-to-one correspondence by passing out materials such as books, milk cartons, or art supplies to peers in class.

5. The family priority of making friends was not included on Josh's IEP as a behavioral goal for him, but was rather addressed through the development of a circle of friends.
6. During arrival and dismissal times, Josh will independently manage the belongings in his knapsack.
7. The family priority of spending time with friends was not written as an IEP goal but was addressed by staff and family working to get Josh enrolled in the after-school latch-key program and one town recreation department sport each semester.
8. In cooperation with a peer, Josh will work in the school's recycling program 3 days per week.

Some readers may wonder why the program development process attends to the development of annual goals before a discussion of how the student will participate in the regular education curriculum. Isn't this antithetical to the notion of inclusion? Do we risk paying so much attention to the "trees" that we lose sight of the "forest"? The authors also admit that the process of developing students' IEP's sometimes seems cumbersome, especially when we are promoting fewer differences between typical students and students with disabilities relative to curriculum and participation. When students are preschool or elementary age, we agree that it might make sense for the determination of annual goals and short-term objectives to come after a discussion of how the student will participate in the regular education classroom and if or how curriculum will be adapted for an individual learning style. All preschool and elementary age students—students who are typical or those with disabilities—usually partake of the whole curriculum. Everyone goes to gym, everyone has language arts instruction, everyone has science instruction. Students with disabilities are simply included in all of those activities and lessons. In this situation, the determination of a focus (goals and objectives) for the student's learning might be done by reviewing the general curriculum goals for all students and picking and choosing areas of emphasis for the student with the disability. When teams have tried to do this they have discovered that there are, however, some learning areas relevant to students with disabilities that are "missing" in the general education curriculum, so that they have to add them in later. For some students with severe disabilities, learning outcomes from the general education curriculum may not be expressed with enough variability (e.g., allowing varied means for demonstrating mastery) for the broad range of students identified as having severe disabilities.

Another difficulty in looking first at curriculum before having identified a student's learning priorities is that at the middle and high school levels, all students have choices about which classes they take. All students—those with and without disabilities— should be thinking about their strengths and needs as they are picking classes and extracurricular activities. Perhaps the solution to the dilemmas encountered when trying to intermingle students and curricula from two systems (regular and special) is to reorganize education into one, unified system for all students. Teachers and support staff would no longer have to spend long hours trying to understand each others' idiosyncratic language, teams might have more time to develop individualized learning goals and strategies for every student, and all students might then be able to benefit from the skills of both general and special education support staff (Stainback & Stainback, 1989). In the meantime, the determination of a student's priority learning goals is a necessary, oftentimes frustrating, but potentially helpful way for teams to make informed decisions about course selection, the need for and role of related services support, and criteria for evaluating student progress.

Review of Process Thus Far

To review the process thus far, the following steps have been accomplished:

1. Members of the team have gotten to know the student with the disability through discussion with the student, his family, former teachers, and friends. Perhaps a M.A.P.S. session has been completed so that the team knows the student's likes and dislikes, strengths and needs, and long-range dreams.
2. If necessary, the team has identified any barriers that make inclusion difficult, and team members have taken responsibility for addressing those barriers before the student's first day in the new class or school.
3. The team has acknowledged the importance of friends in the student's life and plans have been made to expand the student's social relationships through encouragement of natural supports and, perhaps, establishment of a formal "circle of friends."

4. The most important learning goals for the student have been identified for the current school year and they have been written as annual goals for the student's IEP.

The next phase of the program development process hones in on the details of the student's program. What will the student do during classroom lessons? What are we expecting the student will learn in those lessons? What kind of support will be needed? What is the role of the various teaching and support staff in the process? How will we know if things are going well?

Step 5: Specify Participation in the Regular Education Curriculum and Typical School Routines and Revise Needs for Support

Even before the student enters the classroom, teams have found it very helpful to develop a "participation matrix" to guide teachers and other staff during the first few weeks of school. A matrix was developed for Josh, the 10-year-old 5th grader and is the result of the team's initial brainstorming about how he will participate in each class and school activity (see Figure 2–1). Although there are many different kinds of matrices, this one places the student's priority learning goals on the left-hand axis and lists his daily schedule across the top of the matrix. The team then describes in general how the student is expected to participate in each class, given what's important to learn.

As one examines this preliminary participation matrix, the richness of the regular education classroom environment is apparent. There are probably hundreds of opportunities for students to learn important skills and attitudes, even if they aren't targeted for instruction. At the time this matrix was developed, Josh's team decided that some classes just didn't afford opportunities for him to learn certain IEP skills. Those are designed by N/A—not applicable. TBD (to be determined) indicates that the team felt as if there might be opportunities for him to learn the skill within a class or environment, but that they needed to think more about it, after Josh had been included in 5th grade for a few weeks. Strategies to conduct those problem-solving deliberations are presented in Chapters 3 and 5, which deal with curriculum modification for meaningful participation.

If the team were to try to write short-term objectives for each goal at this point in the planning process, they would be frustrated for a number of reasons: (a) the team has not yet observed the student's participation within the regular classroom or other school activities, so they have not yet had a chance to gather baseline information on the student's current level of performance; (b) objectives need to be written for implementation within the normal ebb and flow of the classroom, given the unique style of the general education teacher, the behavior of other students in the classroom, and so forth; and (c) some objectives should be written so that they can be addressed across many environments, and the team has not yet identified nor observed the student in those places.

Therefore, developing short-term objectives and specific ideas for teaching must wait until the student is included in the regular classroom, which may not be until the following September. By this time, all team members will have observed the student and obtained meaningful baseline data on the students' performance within the classroom in preparation for estimating specific criteria for each short-term objective. This process should begin the first day that the student is in the regular class and should be thought of as an ongoing evaluation of the student's progress and the effectiveness of instruction. In all our years of consulting to New Hampshire schools, we have seen fewer than a handful of IEPs truly utilized as living documents. Teams should constantly evaluate how students are doing in their classes and the list of short-term objectives should be frequently amended and expanded to reflect how students are changing. This is a radical departure from the way that IEPs have been utilized in the past. Formerly, goals and objectives were written at the beginning of the year, progress reports were issued a few times during the year to describe how the student had progressed relative to the original projections, and a year-end summary report indicated how well the student did relative to what the team projected (guessed) nearly a year previously. How much more useful it would be if short-term objectives were revised frequently without going through a lengthy IEP meeting, so that parents and team members could see a running record of how the student learned in various situations, what experiences led to spurts of learning, and which seemed to slow down progress. When parents in New Hampshire have been asked for permission to use the IEP in this way, they have been thrilled to think that their child's teachers were continually reviewing how he or she was

Schedule/Goal	Arrival	Writing	Gym	Snack	Lang. Arts	Recycling	Lunch	Recess	Science	Exploratories	Dismissal
Make choices	Walk in with friends of own choosing	Choose topic from communication book or photo album	As captain, choose team members	Choose who to sit next to for snack	Choose book	N/A	Choose entree for hot lunch	Choose equipment to play on or kids to hang around with	Choose station and project to work on	Choose colors for painting sets for play	Choose who to sit next to on bus
Sustain interactions	Extend greeting to teacher, peers	Maintain attention to peer during conferencing time	N/A	Have conversations with peers during snack	When teacher asks question, use communication book or gestures to answer	Communicate with peers while doing job	If server doesn't understand choice, continue to indicate selection	N/A	Maintain focus on group project and answer students' questions	Communicate with peers during play rehearsals	N/A
Learn school routine	Walk with kids to lockers	Get journal from files	Line up on blue line at beginning of class	Get snack from lunch crate before going back in classroom	TBD	Crush cans and toss in bins with peer model	Get silverware at beginning of line	Line up in correct place at end of recess	Find science kits in storage closet	Walk to auditorium unassisted	Go to correct bus at end of day
One-to-one correspondence	N/A	Pass out journals to group	Pass out pinnies to teammates	Pass out milk to students	TBD	N/A	N/A	N/A	Pass out kits to each team	N/A	N/A

Schedule/Goal	Arrival	Writing	Gym	Snack	Lang. Arts	Recycling	Lunch	Recess	Science	Exploratories	Dismissal
Spend leisure time with friends	Walk to school with friends	Conference with classmates	Have fun!	Sit with friends at snack	N/A	N/A	Sit with friends at lunch table	Play organized game or just hang out	N/A	Have fun working on play	Walk to bus with friends
Manage belongings	Hang backpack in locker; bring needed materials into classroom	Locate journal in file and bring to writing corner	Change into sneakers before gym, if necessary	Get snack from lunch box in lunch crate; put thermos back in lunch box and return to crate	N/A	N/A	Remember to give lunch ticket to check-out worker	N/A	Locate science notebook in desk	N/A	Remember to put lunch box and other school supplied in knapsack, and bring home at end of day
Make friends	Walk to school with same group every day	Build relationships from shared experiences	Have fun!	Sit with friends during snack	N/A	Invite recycling teammates for weekend play	Sit with friends	Play games and hang out	N/A	Attend rehearsals and cast party	Sit with friends on bus
Do a school job	N/A	N/A	N/A	N/A	N/A	Work at recycling first semester; another job second semester	N/A	N/A	N/A	N/A	N/A

FIGURE 2-1

Matrix of opportunities for Josh to learn IEP goals in 5th grade classes and general school environments.

Key: N/A Indicates that at the time, the team didn't think that the class afforded an opportunity for Josh to learn this skill

TBD Indicates that team identified the need to do more brainstorming about this class after Josh had been in school a few weeks learning, and they have given their wholehearted permission for the team to make frequent adjustments to the IEP (W. Wansart, personal communication, January 1, 1993).

Step 6. Write Short-term Objectives Based on Classroom Observations, Team Evaluations, and Discrepancy Analyses

There are two interrelated activities which provide team members with information needed to write meaningful short-term objectives. During the first few weeks a student is included in a regular class, various team members should observe in those classes and use team meeting time to identify possible problems, identify teachers' need for assistance or training, and to provide a context for more specific evaluation activities. The second activity is to conduct environmentally based or curriculum-referenced assessments which will establish baseline information on skill performance, the student's response to various kinds of instruction, and the discrepancy between current performance and the skills the student needs to be as involved as typical students (Brown, Shiraga, York, Zanaga, & Rogan, 1984). Chapter 4 discusses strategies for conducting communication skill assessment within regular class and school activities and environments.

Classroom Observations

To begin the ongoing process of developing and revising short-term objectives and teaching plans, one or more staff members should conduct observations during the first few weeks of school in several of the student's classes and other school and community settings for the purpose of: (1) developing an overall picture of the student's participation in instructional and noninstructional activities; (2) determining if opportunities exist for the student to work on all of his goals; (3) documenting what learning styles and strategies the student relies on to gain new information and solve problems; (4) assessing the quality of the student's interaction with peers in structured and non-structured situations; (5) determining how comfortable and skilled teachers are at involving students and providing instruction (to identify need for teacher training or support); (6) developing curriculum modification ideas; and (7) determining if the student (and the teacher) is receiving enough support.

A form and guidelines for collecting this general information has been developed by Jorgensen (1991).

The observation conducted in Josh's 5th grade class typifies the kind of information gleaned from an environmental observation such as this, and is presented in Table 2–4 (Jorgensen, 1992). Each team member receives a copy of the observation and it can trigger problem-solving activities that can be conducted as a team during weekly planning meetings or by individual team members who work on their own and then bring ideas to the whole team for reaction.

An analysis of the information collected from the in-class observation follows.

Overall Picture of Josh's Participation in 5th Grade

Josh's day looks like a nice balance between time spent on academic tasks and time to socialize with friends. The most unstructured times of the day provide rich opportunities for Josh to develop the communication and social skills that his family sees as a priority. The academic times of the day are underutilized as instructional time for Josh. He is marginally involved, especially in writing and science.

Are Josh's Learning Goals Being Met?

Josh has ample opportunity to learn new skills by observing other students, by repeated practice within familiar routines, and from some direct instruction from support personnel when they are immediately available to Josh within the classroom. Additional attention to some of Josh's other learning goals (one-to-one correspondence, and work routines) should be addressed or the staff should reassess if those skills are a priority this year.

Description of Josh's Learning Style and Approaches to Problem-solving

Josh uses observation and modeling of other students in his approach to solving unfamiliar problems. If there is not a model available for the appropriate behavior or response, he looks expectantly at others and waits for assistance. Teaching should focus on providing a peer model for Josh and if prompting is necessary, using the least intrusive prompt and fading back as soon as possible.

TABLE 2–4
Josh's day at school

Time	Class/Activity	What Does Josh Do?	Support
8:00	Children are off to school by car, bus, walking.	Josh's mother drops him off in front of school.	Mom drives Josh and two other neighborhood boys.
8:05	Kids play on playground before school bell rings Josh's buddies are throwing a ball against the outside wall of the school.	Josh and friends walk over to side of building—Josh is just standing with the other boys—He acknowledges their greetings with a smile and an excited giggle.	Other students walk with Josh—they slow their pace a little so Josh can keep up.
8:15	School bell rings—kids rush into school.	Josh looks toward the bell and walks along.	No support necessary—he knows routine.
8:20	Kids hang up coats in lockers in hall, get lunches and books out of knapsacks.	Josh gets to the right area but then just stands in front of lockers.	Kid next to Josh says "Hang your coat up, Josh." Opens locker for him, takes his hand and helps him unzip coat. Hangs his coat in locker. Says, "close your locker and bring your knapsack."

Time			
8:25	Students put their lunch boxes in crate and go to the writing folder boxes—they get their own and go to their desks.	Josh gives the locker door a push, picks up knapsack and follows friend into the room.	Teacher says, "Hi Josh" and gently puts Josh's hands down. Says, "Let's put your lunch away and get your writing." He walks with Josh to where the lunch boxes are kept. Asks Josh, "Where does this go?" and prompts Josh to put his lunch box under the picture of his lunch box.
		Josh goes up to teacher and takes his hands—smiles and shakes his hands up and down.	
		Josh finds the picture of his lunch box—alternates his gaze from his lunch box to the picture and sets it on the counter.	
		Josh finds his folder and sits down at his desk.	Teacher says, "Matt, would you please help Josh find his folder—just have him find the one with his picture on it. Thanks."

TABLE 2-4
(continued)

Time	Class/Activity	What Does Josh Do?	Support
	Teacher says, "All right, let's try to get some writing in before announcements."		
8:40	Announcements come on.	He listens and looks at the P.A. speaker.	None needed.
	Pledge of Allegiance.	Josh stands with everyone else—looks around when Pledge is recited—puts his hand on his heart.	Student next to Josh motions for Josh to put his hand on his heart.
8:45	Students return to writing.	He looks through his scrapbook and points to pictures of his Boy Scout Troop on a recent camp out.	Two students go up to Josh and say, "Let's go over to the reading corner." They all go behind a partition and sit on a small loveseat. Josh is between the boys. They read their journals and offer suggestions to each

Time			
			other, ask questions. They talk with Josh about the camping trip and ask him to point to various people he knows.
9:10	Students get into pairs and share their reading. Teacher comes around and asks each pair about their journal entries.	Josh reads with another pair of students.	Students come over to Josh and ask him about the pictures. They share their writing with him.
9:25	Students put their writing folders away and get ready for gym.	Josh takes his folder up to the file boxes—he lays it on the shelf. He tries to put folder in box but it won't go in.	One student says, "Time to put our writing away— can you put yours in the front of the box?" Student puts it in for him.
9:30	Students get up and leave for gym.	Josh gets up and walks with group.	No support needed.
9:35	Students run around the gym five times.	Josh bounce-walks with the gym teacher—he gets about 1/4 of the way around one lap then stops and watches rest of class.	Gym teacher keeps up friendly banter as he sort of jogs in place next to Josh.

TABLE 2–4
(continued)

Time	Class/Activity	What Does Josh Do?	Support
9:40	Students sit in a circle as teacher describes game called "Freddy Kruger"—modern version of "Red Rover."	Josh sits with group but occasionally flops onto his back and rolls from side to side.	No support needed.
9:45	One student in the middle is "Freddy"—he tries to capture helpers as class runs across Freddy's space.	He plays just like other students—laughs and runs wrong way sometimes. Tries to catch other kids because he became a helper when "Freddy" tagged him.	Kids form a protective circle around Josh and sort of shepherd him across gym floor. No support needed.
10:10	Gym class over—students line up for a drink at the fountain.	Josh lines up for a drink too. He tries to push button—can't push it hard enough. He drinks when water comes on. Gets pretty wet.	Peer puts his hand over Josh's and pushes so that water comes out.

Time	Activity	Josh	Support
10:15	Class walks back to their room.	Josh walks with other students.	No assistance needed.
10:18	Snack	Josh carries his chips and juice pack to his desk. Josh eats his chips and drinks from his juice pack.	Another student helps Josh get his snack out of his knapsack. He says, "Let's go eat our snack." Student opens Josh's chips and puts straw in juice pack.
10:25	Language arts—continued. Students working in 4 groups—2 groups writing a persuasive speech for and against mandatory locker searches for drugs; 1 group making a collage showing alternative activities to do instead of using drugs and alcohol—"Healthy Lifestyle Choices"; 1 group is putting together a display for the foyer on the dangers of using drugs.	Josh is working with the group that is making the collage—his role is to choose scenes for the collage and paste them on the poster board.	Speech-language pathologist comes in to work with the group Josh is in. SLP shows the other students how to give Josh a choice from among two that the students have cut out. Enters into discussion with students about their choices. Role plays, "What would you do it someone offered you drugs? What should Josh do?"

TABLE 2–4
(continued)

Time	Class/Activity	What Does Josh Do?	Support
11:00	Math Students are working on multiplying and dividing fractions.	Josh leaves the room at this time to work in the school's recycling business.	Two students from the the 8th grade come to pick up Josh and they go down to the cafeteria.
11:05	Math	Josh and two friends sort paper, cans, and plastic ware.	Friends guide Josh to put the cans in the can bin one by one, and the plastic ware in the plastic bin.
11:45	Class is finished with math and they have a current events discussion.	Josh is done with job and comes back to the classroom. Josh goes to the boy's room to have his Attends changed.	Recycling pals walk Josh back to classroom. Paraprofessional meets Josh there and walks with him to the boy's room. There is a screened off corner where she changes his Attends.
11:55	Class still discussing the Middle East situation.	Josh returns to classroom and sits at his desk.	No support needed. Paraprofessional

Time			
		He listens to the class discussion.	walks him back to class.
12:00	Lunchtime Some students go through the lunch line, others bring cold lunch and go directly to a table.	Josh eats cold lunch. He has a sandwich, chips, and gets milk in the line.	Lunch workers help Josh get his milk carton. They know that his milk ticket is in his shirt pocket and help him get it out.
12:30	Lunch is over and kids go outside for recess. Some kids play ball games some are using climbing apparatus, others talking.	Josh walks out with friend. He sees kids he knows and goes up to them. Group of girls talks and walks with him around the blacktop.	Friend waits while Josh throws bag away, then they all just walk outside together. Friend goes to other group.
12:45	Bell rings and recess is over. Kids go inside the building.	Josh wanders over to the equipment, picks up the pea stone and plays with it.	Recess monitor goes up to Josh and says, "Josh, it's time to go inside now. You are in Mr. Carney's room, aren't you?"
		He smiles at Monitor but walks farther away from the school entrance.	Monitor takes him by the arm and talks to him as they walk into the school.
		He goes with Monitor.	

TABLE 2–4
(continued)

Time	Class/Activity	What Does Josh Do?	Support
12:55	Science		
	The teacher is continuing the unit on electricity. Teacher asks kids to get out their texts and follow along as he reads the definition of the two types of circuits. Teacher then draws diagrams of the two types of circuits on the board. Task is to set up both circuits and to see which arrangement will light more wattage.	Josh will work with his small group to build a parallel and a series circuit. Objective is for Josh to hand a student various materials that the student points to. Josh is in charge of the materials.	The students in his group will help Josh do the physical parts of the task.

The teacher has six trays of materials. He hands a tray to a student from each group. Puts tray in front of Josh. |
| 1:05 | | Students work in groups to put together circuits. They are discussing what they think will happen, trying to explain what does happen. | Josh hands materials to students—he doesn't know names of objects, but responds to the request. | Students ask, "Josh give me the light bulb, please" while pointing to the object. |

Time			
1:20	Teacher directs each group to write up one lab report in a cooperative fashion. Students assume various roles in the group. Tells them they have 20 minutes to finish.	Josh's job is to put all materials back into tray and take tray back to the cabinet.	He is prompted to do that by various students as they engage in the discussion.
		Josh is the timekeeper and is supposed to tell the class when time is up.	Another student sets the timer and puts it in front of Josh. Teacher says, "Josh will tell us when time is up."
		Josh sits with his group as they discuss. His attention wanders, but he seems fine.	Students periodically ask, "Is our time up Josh? How many minutes left?" They point to the number on the timer and say, "Ten minutes left, Josh."
	Groups know the parts of the report and work together to dictate their observations to the student who is doing the writing.		
1:40	Time's up. Teacher says, "We only have time for one group to share their report. Group number 2, why don't you come up to the front of the room. Now, first tell me who took what	Josh is named as the timekeeper.	

TABLE 2-4
(continued)

Time	Class/Activity	What Does Josh Do?	Support
	role? Who's going to read the report?" Student reads report. Teacher asks each student a question about their observations, conclusions.	Josh stands with his group as they read report.	No support needed.
1:50	Exploratory Period During the last period of the day, students have a choice of receiving tutoring, working on homework, or participating in special activities like school newspaper, chess club, tai chi, and so on. Typical students may do special activities 2 times per week.	Josh goes to work on the set of a play that the drama club is doing. Josh is painting sets. Working on sustaining interactions with other students, making choices, making friends, spending leisure time with friends.	OT picks Josh up and walks to the art room with him and five other students from Josh's classroom.
		Josh does special activities 5 times per week.	OT works right alongside set-painting crew.

Students are talking, gossiping.

Josh chooses colors to paint with.

When Josh tries to paint, he can't really hold the brush tightly enough. OT says, "Guys, this isn't working for Josh. Do you have any ideas?" One girl says, "When Josh plays drums in music class, he has some kind of white thing wrapped around the sticks. Would that help?" OT says, "Maybe. I'll go to my office and see if I have any more of that stuff."

While OT is gone, a girl helps Josh hold the paintbrush to steady it. OT comes back and wraps foam around a paintbrush.

TABLE 2–4
(continued)

Time	Class/Activity	What Does Josh Do?	Support
2:20	First bell rings for dismissal. Other students quickly wash brushes and rush back to their classrooms. Students get their books, knapsacks, lunch boxes, coats.	Josh can't help clean up because he takes longer going back to the classroom. He doesn't like being rushed and protests.	OT walks him back to his classroom. She runs into the classroom and asks the teacher, "Does Josh need to bring anything home tonight?" Teacher speaks above the noise, "Just his knapsack."
2:30	Final bell rings for dismissal. Kids stream out and line up for the bus.	Josh doesn't have his coat on yet.	OT helps him put on his coat, knapsack and rushes him out the door. She asks several students "Does anybody know which bus Josh is supposed to ride on?" Principal is standing in foyer and says, "Bus 16". OT takes him to correct line and he gets on bus.

Quality and Quantity of Peer Interactions

Josh has lots of peer interactions during the day, but conversations are fleeting. Students who talk to Josh generally ask him one sentence questions (e.g. "How was your weekend?") or provide instruction to him ("Here's the way you open that milk carton"). Students don't talk to him in baby talk, but there is a sense from their conversations that their relationship with him is confined to the school day. The team should step up efforts to find a Big Brother to accompany Josh to recreation department Saturday activities.

Curriculum Modification and Teaching Strategies

Josh's involvement in the academic times of the day is minimal. The team needs to brainstorm how Josh can be more meaningfully involved in writing time, in math (although the recycling task is enjoyable, meaningful, and includes students without disabilities, it does remove him from his own class), and in science. Chapter 3 addresses curriculum modification in depth.

Staff Comfort and Skill at Providing Instruction

All staff who interact with Josh seem comfortable around him and their style of instruction and assistance fits nicely within the general atmosphere of his classroom. People treat Josh respectfully and seem to have an attitude of "pitching in when necessary" to provide support to him when there isn't another staff person around. Josh doesn't receive very much direct instruction throughout the day, except when related service staff come into class to work with his group.

Supports Josh Currently Receives which Facilitate His Participation

Josh's most effective supports are currently his peers. He receives some direct support from his regular class teachers, from the SLP, a paraprofessional, and from the occupational therapist (OT).

Writing Short-term Objectives

Most special education professionals have written objectives that sound like this: "During snack, library time, and the lunch line and given a verbal cue 'What do you want, John?' he will make a choice 75% of the time from among 3 concrete objects placed within his visual field, as measured by daily observations." Do we seriously believe that regular classroom teachers will identify with the way this objective is written, given the demands for data gathering? Is there another way to write short-term objectives so that they are meaningful to everyone on the team, so that they actually reflect the reality of what students have learned, and so that they can be modified over time as students change?

Teams face a number of serious roadblocks in trying to write short-term objectives that are meaningful, authentic and durable over time. The first is that professionals from different disciplines were taught to write objectives differently. Second, many school districts try to standardize the way their IEPs look and proscribe the way that objectives are written. Third, there is a common misconception about what needs to be included in short-term objectives from a regulatory and legal standpoint.

According to Giangreco, Cloninger, & Iverson (1993, p. 63), "writing short-term objectives is a refining process whereby generally stated goals are broken down into a sequence of small steps. . . Generally, objectives include three distinct components: 1) conditions, 2) behavior, and 3) criteria." Because the C.O.A.C.H. process requires that the team develop a unified set of discipline-free annual goals, there is an opportunity within the short-term objectives to target the cognitive, communicative, behavioral or movement aspects of a goal, depending on the student's needs. C.O.A.C.H. suggests many components that can be addressed through short-term objectives including: (a) desensitization/ increasing tolerance; (b) acquiring core skills; (c) preparation for the activity; (d) tempo or rate; (e) self-monitoring; (f) termination of the behavior; (g) safety aspects of participating in the activity; (h) communicative aspects of the behavior; (i) indication of choice or preference; (j) generalization across setting, cues, materials, individuals; (k) quality of the performance of the behavior.

Given the almost unlimited choices for expressing short-term objectives, it becomes clear that families and team members must accept that the IEP is only a subset of all possible learning outcomes, not an exhaustive summary of the student's total educational plan. Team members must be willing to forgo the volumes of communication goals, the lists of leisure skills, the myriad of fine motor skills that might be targeted given unlimited time and resources, and instead focus on a small number of really essential skills that will promote the student's inclusion and learning in the current school year.

One of the most common misconceptions is that behavior and criteria must be expressed using numbers and percentages. Rhodes and Dudly-Marling (1986) summarize the misuse of behaviorally written objectives:

> Behavioral objectives are well motivated. They presume to ensure maximally efficient instruction by focusing on well-defined, easily achievable "building blocks" of learning. But they depend on a technology that does not exist. Precise descriptions of cognitive, social, and linguistic behavior . . . are not possible and probably not desirable. Behavioral objectives trivialize learning, seriously underestimate the potential of learners . . . and strip away the meaningfulness of what is presented to students. (p. 67)

Rhodes and Dudly-Marling suggest a way of writing objectives that is consistent with a more holistic way of looking at students' lives and learning, that still covers accountability and fulfills legal responsibilities. Continuing with the example of Josh, meaningful, yet measureable objectives for several of his annual goals are presented in Table 2–5.

TABLE 2–5
Examples of annual goals and short-term objectives for Josh

Goal: Within real-life situations such as choosing food in the lunchroom, selecting books in the library, or picking friends to be on his team in gym, Josh will make a choice from among 3 offerings.

Objective
When presented with a natural cue and a gestural prompt across various settings (e.g., the server asking him what he wants for hot lunch and if he doesn't choose, the server will point to the various choices), Josh will point to a choice (from among 3) within the time limit given other students. This will be measured by observations across at least three settings and by interviewing peers and teachers.

Goal: When talking with a responsive peer, Josh will take three conversational turns using his communication book or natural gestures.

Objective
During informal conversation or buddy-reading in the classroom, Josh will maintain his interest in a book or a picture from home by answering

at least three questions posed by a peer. The SLP will observe in the classroom once a week in different settings to evaluate Josh's progress.

Goal: Josh will demonstrate an understanding of one-to-one correspondence by passing out materials such as books, milk cartons, or art supplies to peers in class.

Objective
When accompanied by a peer who cues Josh by counting, "One, two, three, four," Josh will pass out materials to peers in class, with accuracy up to 10. This objective will be evaluated by interviewing peers and observing Josh in class.

Goal: During arrival and dismissal times, Josh will independently manage the belongings in his knapsack.

Objective
On arrival at school, Josh will independently unpack his knapsack at his locker. He will put his lunch box in the lunch box crate, carry his books and notebooks to his desk, hang his knapsack in his locker, and make his way to his seat by the time the first bell rings. This objective will be evaluated by having a peer make a daily yes/no check on a chart kept in Josh's desk and by having his mother do the same at home.

Goal: In cooperation with a peer, Josh will work in the school's recycling program 3 days per week.

Objective
Josh will independently participate in an assembly-line can crushing process with verbal reminders from peers. The team will be evaluated by the assistant principal about whether they meet their quota of cans each week. Evaluation will be done by asking students and by having a paraprofessional observe once a week for the second term and count the number of verbal reminders that Josh needs.

■□ SUMMARY

This chapter has outlined some new strategies for getting to know students, identifying barriers to their successful inclusion, facilitating peer relationships, identifying what learning objectives are most important to focus on for a current school year, and outlining some initial ideas for how the student will participate in a regular class.

The next steps in the process presented include (a) developing creative curriculum modification ideas for involving students in classroom lessons and activities that focus on their learning priorities, (b) specifying the role of teachers and support staff in the process, (c) identifying the evaluation criteria for measuring the student's learning and our teaching.

■□ REFERENCES

Biklen, D. (Ed.). (1985). *The complete school: Strategies for effective mainstreaming.* New York: Columbia University, Teacher's College Press.

Brown, L., Shiraga, B., York, J., Zanella, K., & Rogan, K. (1984). *The discrepancy analysis technique in programs for students with severe handicaps.* Madison: University of Wisconsin-Madison and Madison Metropolitan School District.

Forest, M., & O'Brien, J. (1989). *Action for inclusion.* Toronto, Ontario: Centre for Integrated Education, Frontier College.

Giangreco, M., Cloninger, C., & Iverson, V. (1993). *Choosing options and accommodations for children (C.O.A.C.H.): A guide to planning inclusive education.* Baltimore: Paul H. Brookes Publishing Co.

Jorgensen, C. (1991). *What to look for when observing classroom lessons or typical school routines in order to identify participation opportunities for students with severe disabilities.* Durham: Institute on Disability, University of New Hampshire.

Jorgensen, C. (1992). Natural supports in inclusive schools: Curricular and teaching strategies. In J. Nisbet (Ed.), *Natural supports in school, at work, and in the community for people with severe disabilities* (pp. 179–215). Baltimore: Paul H. Brookes Publishing Co.

Mount, B. (1987). *Personal futures planning: Finding directions for change.* Ann Arbor: University of Michigan Dissertation Information Service.

New Hampshire Developmental Disabilities Council. (1989). *Promises to keep: Supporting persons with developmental disabilities, their families and community in the 1990's.* Concord, NH: Developmental Disabilities Council.

Nisbet, J., & Hagner, D. (1988). Natural supports in the workplace: A reexamination of supported employment. *Journal of the Association for Persons with Severe Handicaps, 13,* 260-267.

Pearpoint, J. (1991). *From behind the piano: The building of Judith Snow's unique circle of friends.* Toronto: Inclusion Press.

Perske, R., & Perske, M. (1988). *Circles of friends: People with disabilities and their friends enrich the lives of one another.* Nashville: Abingdon Press.

Rhodes, L., & Dudly-Marling, C. (1988). *Readers and writers with a difference: A holistic approach to teaching learning disabled and remedial students.* Portsmouth, NH: Heinemann Press.

Schaffner, C. B., & Buswell, B. E. (1991). *Opening doors: Strategies for including all students in regular education.* Colorado Springs: PEAK Parent Center, Inc.

Sizer, T. (1992). *Horace's school. Redesigning the American high school.* Boston: Houghton Mifflin Co.

Stainback, S., Stainback, W., & Forest, M. (Eds.). (1989). *Educating all students in the mainstream of regular education.* Baltimore: Paul H. Brookes Publishing Co.

Strully, J.L., & Strully, C.F. (1989). Friendships as an educational goal. In S. Stainback, W. Stainback, & M. Forest (Eds.), *Educating all students in the mainstream of regular education* (pp. 59-68). Baltimore: Paul H. Brookes Publishing Co.

Tashie, C., Shapiro-Barnard, C., Schuh, M., Jorgensen, C., Dillon, A., & Nisbet, J. (1993). *Changes in lattitude, changes in attitude: The role of the inclusion facilitator.* Durham, NH: Institute on Disability, University of New Hampshire.

Vandercook, T., York, J., & Forest, M. (1989). The McGill action planning system (M.A.P.S.): A strategy for building the vision. *Journal of the Association for Persons with Severe Handicaps, 14,* 205-215.

Modifying the Curriculum and Short-Term Objectives to Foster Inclusion

Cheryl M. Jorgensen

■ INTRODUCTION

In Chapter 2 we described (a) strategies for getting to know students in ways that will enhance the likelihood of their successful inclusion, (b) the rationale supporting and some practical ideas for facilitating circles of friends and natural supports for students who are included, (c) a model for identifying the most important learning goals and accompanying short-term objectives for a student's individualized education plan (IEP), and (d) the necessity of conducting regular classroom observations to form a context for ongoing discussion of how academic lessons and other school activities can be modified to enable students to derive meaning from them.

This chapter presents strategies for including students with severe disabilities in regular classroom and school activities, many examples of student participation and short-term objectives (displayed in the boxes interspersed throughout the chapter), and guidelines for using an instructional planning form for recording both IEP objectives and general classroom participation. At the end of the chapter, the entire instructional planning and curriculum modification process will be illustrated through the example of Josh's (introduced in Chapter 2) science class.

■□ THREE MORE SCENARIOS

As you read the three scenarios which introduce this chapter, think about how the teachers in each situation are using the best practices presented in Chapters 1 and 2. Focus on their commitment to keeping students with severe disabilities alongside their peers in academic classes and during informal classroom activities. Take notice of the curriculum development and modification strategies that they used to assure that students are not only physically present in classes but are participating and learning as well. Following presentation of these representative scenarios a comprehensive discussion of curriculum modification and short-term objectives will be presented along with additional examples of students of all ages.

Golden Brook Elementary School

Three teachers from the Windham School District started "The Breakfast Club" as a way to integrate the teaching of functional living skills with academic instruction in a way that would benefit all the students in the third grade classes. Each Monday students plan the breakfast they will sell to teachers on Thursday; they find a recipe, check their inventory, estimate shopping expenses, and make a shopping list. On Tuesday, a small group of students shop for the needed ingredients. Students without disabilities have one opportunity each semester to go shopping and students with functional goals on their IEPs shop every week. On Wednesday, students compare actual expenses with their estimated expenses and determine how much they will have to charge for each item in order to meet their financial goals. Advertising posters are made and posted around the school. On Thursday, students make and sell the baked goods to teachers and other staff. On Friday, students figure their profits from their Thursday sales and graph the current week's profits against past weeks' profits.

Students gain specific skills in the areas of (a) math (profit margins, metric conversions, proportional recipe amount increases, comparative price shopping, basic operations, word problems); (b) reading and language arts (communication skills, creating posters and flyers, advertising); (c) science (nutritional values, measurement); (d) social studies (community involvement, salesmanship, cooperation with other classmates); and (e) computer technology (graphing sales and profits). Stocks are sold to parents and teachers, monthly dividends returned to stock holders, and a "Breakfast Club Recipe Book" has been sold to make additional money for the "corporation."

Hanover Street School

Jordan attended 4th grade along with the other 9-year-olds at his school in Lebanon, NH. His educational goals did not include traditional academics. Because Jordan was blind and had severe cerebral palsy and mental retardation, his school goals focused on his ability to indicate choices, have increased control over his environment and schedule, enjoy increased participation in shared activities with his friends, and maintain a healthy body. Every day after recess, Jordan's teacher read to her students from a chapter book. The students gathered in a cozy carpeted meeting area; some children sat cross-legged, some relaxed in bean bag chairs, and others sprawled on the floor. Jordan lay down in the center of the meeting area and while the teacher was reading, children gently massaged his head and shoulders while others did slow stretching exercises with his arms and legs. Jordan got valuable relaxation time while listening to the soothing voice of his teacher and feeling the gentle touch of his friends.

Souhegan High School

Dave, an 18-year-old high school senior who has developmental disabilities, was enrolled in the senior seminar class at Souhegan

High School in Amherst, NH. Each senior must complete a comprehensive research project presented to the student body and community as a sample exhibition of what the student has learned throughout 4 years in high school. Last year was Dave's first year as a member of a regular class in a nonsegregated school. Based on consultation with his mentor and his senior seminar teacher, he selected fishing as the focus of his senior project. He visited the New Hampshire Fish and Game Department and gathered pictures and brochures depicting various aspects of commercial and sport fishing in the state that were displayed on a poster, he interviewed several family friends talking about their fishing experiences and produced a videotape of their stories, and exhibited several types of flys that he had tied. The previous summer Dave had worked at a local fish hatchery, supported by funds from his school district (his "extended year program"), the state Job Corps, and the local developmental services agency.

■◻ WHY MODIFY CURRICULUM?

We can safely conclude that the teachers and students involved in these examples have a high regard for the contributions that students with disabilities can make to a classroom and to a school. Their efforts show that they value inclusion and believe that when classrooms include students with many kinds of differences, learning opportunities for all students can be enriched. The teachers in these scenarios have taken the time to get to know the learning styles and priorities of their students and have used their creativity to structure lessons that will be interesting to the entire class and at the same time meet the specific learning needs of individual students. How did these teachers come to think about teaching in a way that included the needs of all the students in their classes? The first step for many of these teachers was to acknowledge that instruction needs to be adapted to the learning needs and styles of all students in the class, not just those with severe disabilities. Effective teachers realize that you can't teach a class of 30 students using one instructional methodology. They realize that all students have unique learning styles and the best way to ensure that students learn is to use different teaching styles. This means varying how information is presented and allowing students options for demonstrating what they have learned.

> Marcus is a 6th grader who has cerebral palsy, is visually impaired, and has mental retardation. In one English class assignment, the students were expected to read a variety of fables and proverbs, write one of their own and do a related illustration. Marcus worked with another student to complete this assignment. Both boys went to the library and checked out several books of fables. Marcus' peer slowly thumbed through the books, asking Marcus to express a preference for the illustrations that accompanied the stories. When Marcus narrowed his choices to one favorite fable, his friend read it to him out loud, and then went with him to the main office to photocopy the picture. Marcus glued the picture onto construction paper, wrote his name on the top, and turned it in as his assignment. Marcus' peer worked on his own fable alongside Marcus and read him various drafts of his original fable.
>
> The learning objectives that Marcus worked on in this lesson included interacting with peers, looking at pictures in a book for leisure, turning one page at a time, operating a photocopier, learning one-to-one correspondence, and following directions.

■ THREE KINDS OF CURRICULUM MODIFICATION

Depending on the school and the classroom, curriculum modification is accomplished through on-the-spot creative problem solving, through regularly scheduled meetings where upcoming lessons and units are discussed, and on a school-wide basis by all teachers who are restructuring curriculum to be adaptive for every learner. Brief descriptions of these types of curriculum modification are given, followed by a comprehensive presentation of the strategies and values underlying all three models.

On-the-spot Curriculum Modification

Here's a scenario familiar to many support teachers and speech-language pathologists (SLPs). It's 10:10 Tuesday morning and Mr. Robinson departs from the planned lecture on "How We Use Energy in Our Schools and Communities." He decides to take his class on a short walk through the school to survey all the ways that energy is necessary to make schools operate. None of the support staff knew that this activity was going to happen and it is obvious from the look on the teacher's face that he has just realized that he is not sure how to involve Megan in this activity. He wonders, "Do I need to do something to make sure Megan is involved? Should she bring her communication book with her? Should one of the kids help her negotiate the stairs? How does Megan adapt to a change in routine? Isn't it about time for her to go to the girl's room and attend to her personal hygiene needs? The SLP was scheduled to come into the class to help facilitate small discussion groups. How will she know where the class has gone when she finds an empty classroom? "This scenario illustrates "curriculum modification by the seat of your pants!" Teachers, specialists, and paraprofessionals are required to creatively solve problems like this many times each day, even in schools in which teams have adequate planning time. Because teachers often seize the moment for teaching an important concept, all teachers and support staff need to understand that "on the spot" curriculum modification requires using those regular curriculum modification concepts and strategies that can be implemented quickly, before the opportunity has passed!

Ongoing Team Planning for Upcoming Lessons

If all of us worked in ideal schools, with curriculum designed from the start with all students' participation in mind, curriculum modification would be less complicated. However, in schools still struggling with the philosophy of inclusive education, uncertain about how to modify or adapt lessons so that all students are meaningfully involved, a different approach is needed. In these situations, teams must meet on a regular basis to problem-solve inclusion of particular students. An instructional planning team usually includes a few core members: the classroom teacher, a paraprofessional who might be assigned to a student with severe disabilities, and a support teacher, sometimes referred to as an integration or inclusion facilitator. This core team may meet every day for a few minutes, once a week for an hour or more, or later in the year, on a less frequent basis. Related service staff often set up a rotating schedule so that one specialist attends each meeting, but no one person attends more than a couple of meetings a month. The team's success in designing and achieving creative solutions to curriculum modification questions usually mirrors their attitude towards inclusion and their familiarity or lack of experience with collaborative problem-solving strategies (Giangreco, Cloninger, & Iverson, 1993).

Comprehensive Curriculum Revision

The final type of curriculum modification—planning instruction from the beginning with the diversity of learners in mind—usually occurs in schools that have had several years of experience with inclusion, with everyone from the principal to the teaching assistants commited to developing curriculum that includes all students. This can be thought of as designing inclusive curriculum "from the ground up." If schools have already adopted curricular or instructional philosophies and practices that are inherently adaptive—such as the reading and writing process, cooperative learning, and activity-based science curriculum—students with disabilities can be included more easily.

> Jeffrey uses a wheelchair and needs hand-over-hand assistance to move his hands. During 7th grade home economics, Jeffrey stays in the "cooking" rotation while the other students in his half of the class switch over to sewing at mid-semester. In his small group, students provide the hand-over-hand assistance that enables Jeffrey to measure, pour and mix ingredients, wash dishes, and eat the final product!

■ MAKING THE CURRICULUM MODIFICATION PROCESS ONGOING

When students are included in regular classes and activities, the curriculum modification process should be ongoing. Even if the curriculum is flexible and accommodates different learning styles, it is likely that the regular class teacher will need some assistance in planning how students with severe disabilities can participate. The team will need to know if adapted materials need to be developed ahead of time and if student support will need to be arranged. The steps depicted in Table 3–1 illustrate a process for modifying a particular lesson or an entire curriculum. Each step will be discussed in detail following presentation of the overall process.

At the middle school, all students are involved in a 20-minute "homeroom period" at the end of each day. Teachers and administrators facilitate small group discussions on topics such as peer pressure, nuclear war, dating, and drugs. Before this year, team members thought that Susan could only relate to "concrete objects" and, thus, the SLP didn't include abstract feelings and concepts in Susan's picture book. Other students in her homeroom group decided that she needed a way to communicate with other kids on these topics, so her team has added several new pictures—stranger, drugs, lonely, and party—as a result of her participation in this group.

Old Short-term Objective: When presented with a choice of four Mayer-Johnson symbols by the SLP, Susan will eye gaze toward the requested symbol with 80% accuracy 4 out of 5 sessions.

New Short-term Objective: During homeroom period with her peers, Susan will initiate three conversational turns with peers by eye gazing toward a symbol that is on topic in her communication book for 10 consecutive classes.

TABLE 3–1
Steps for modifying regular class curriculum for students with disabilities

---

1. Get to know the students in the class and the priority learning objectives of the student(s) with severe disabilities.
2. Identify general learning opportunities.
3. Describe the overall goal of the lesson.
4. For students with severe disabilities, ask "How can this student participate in this lesson?"
5. Plan lessons and assign responsibilities for developing materials or adapting the environment.
6. Identify ways for students to cooperate with and support one another.
7. Continue ongoing discussions about upcoming lessons.

Step 1: Get To Know all the Students

All teachers have strategies for getting to know their students. These strategies might involve having students write autobiographies on one of the first days of schools. Students might interview one another for a class newsletter and then write a biographical sketch about their new classmate. Some teachers use new games or other adventure-type activities to get their students working as a team early in the school year. Having students work together on a "ropes course" or doing other getting-to-know-you activities can break down barriers quickly. Some teachers who have students with severe disabilities in their classes deal directly with the issue of differences and diversity throughout the year by using literature that explores these issues or by using the "circle of friends" strategy to build support networks for some or all students in their classes. Regardless of the method, teachers and other team members need to have a good understanding of their students' needs if effective curriculum modification is to occur.

> Bernie is a 15-year-old high school sophomore who has mental retardation. The home economics class he takes is doing a semester on drug and alcohol abuse. One group of students is working on
>
> *continued*

researching the health risks of cigarette smoking. Bernie participates by cutting cigarette advertisements out of magazines to help the group show how the media portrays cigarette smokers.

Old Short-term Objective: Using adapted scissors, Bernie will cut out various shapes maintaining less than a 3/8" margin outside of the cutting line with 80% accuracy for 10 therapy sessions.

New Short-term Objective: During regular art and other academic classes, Bernie will maintain hand flexibility and strength by cutting and pasting magazine pictures to make collages as part of small group projects with peers.

Step 2: Identify Regular Class "Learning Opportunities"

Opportunities for students with disabilities to learn are present in all regular classes and school activities, given the right modifications. When designing a student's schedule and the schedule of support staff, it is helpful to keep in mind that potential learning opportunities can exist in every class, and that students with disabilities benefit from participating in regular classes for reasons other than just the acquisition of IEP skills. There is a broader curriculum—called the implied or unspoken curriculum—that students learn when they are in regular classes (Ford et al., 1989). This unspoken curriculum enriches a student's education, helps the individual learn appropriate social behavior, and maintains the student's presence in the regular class.

Academic Skills

Effective educational strategies for typical students—outcomes-based instruction, process reading and writing, hands-on learning, prescriptive teaching, and cooperative learning—can also be effective for students with disabilities.

Friendships

Friendships between students with disabilities and typical students are more likely to develop and be maintained when students are members of the same class and have opportunities to interact with one another during academic and nonstructured activities. When students are included in regular classes only part-time, there is a risk that they will not be thought of when special activities arise. Friendships between students are based on a history of shared experiences, a perception that students have something in common, and a realistic acknowledgment of one another's gifts and vulnerabilities.

Learning to be Part of a Cooperative Group

When teachers structure their classrooms for cooperation and interdependence, all students are seen as having something to contribute and no one has to lose so another can win. Cooperative learning activities more nearly represent the challenges that people face working with one another in adulthood. We all know that the "smartest" of our colleagues are not necessarily the most successful. Individuals who have people skills and who can work as team members have the most flexibility in the types of jobs they can get and are more likely to succeed in the social aspects of the work world.

Organizational and Process Skills

Every activity—whether it is designed for students working independently, in small groups, or in a large group—has process components. These may include initiating activities, preparing materials, socializing, communicating, and reaching closure. In regular classes, there are literally hundreds of organizational and process demands made on typical students that offer valuable learning opportunities for students with disabilities as well. For these students, the ability to successfully carry out these tasks will have many applications for life at home, on the job, and in the community.

Functional Life Skills

It was once thought that even very young students with disabilities should spend most of the school day out in the community learning functional skills such as how to shop, cross streets, and work. For most students, there are many opportunities to learn functional skills within the context of regular classes and school environments; thus, there is little justification for separating students with disabilities from their peers. Arrival and dismissal times, snacktime and lunch, physical education, high school vocational classes and experiences, classroom and other school jobs, as well as extracurricular activities, all provide opportunities for students to learn life skills. For older students (ages 18–21), their last 3 years of entitled educational services should include the same variety of opportunities which are available to their typical age peers. Their choices should include postsecondary education or specialized vocational training, on-the-job training, volunteer work or community service, with a heavy emphasis on building a system of natural supports for the individual so that their inclusion is not wholly dependent on funding and staff from social service agencies. Learning functional life skills should happen where students live, learn, and work. It is "functional" for a school age child to be part of the neighborhood school; as the student enters young adulthood, it is "functional" to learn to be part of the adult world. We propose adding an important criterion to the definition of a functional skill—it's a skill that a student will need to be a fully participating member of a regular class in his or her home school.

Communication, Movement, and Social Skills

All of us learn "by doing" to communicate, to move, and to interact with others. Students with disabilities should develop their communication, movement, and social skills alongside their peers without disabilities. Schools offer unlimited opportunities for learning these skills. In music and art classes, students gain an appreciation for culture and learn to use their senses. Physical education provides time for fun, teamwork, and learning the habits of a healthy lifestyle. Participation in extracurricular activities not only is good recreation, it helps students develop nonacademic talents and interests and offers opportunities for friendships. After-school jobs and volunteer community service develops adult responsibilities and provides opportunities to contribute.

Special Interests

When students with disabilities are placed in separate classes, their curriculum is sometimes less varied than the one offered by the regular class. Opportunities to participate in science, foreign language, social studies, fine arts and applied arts (home economics and industrial arts) can lead to the development of lifelong leisure and vocational interests for students with disabilities.

George is a 4th-grade student in a New Hampshire elementary school. To fulfill the state history curricular requirement, all the students must do a year-long, 20-page report. For his report, George develops a "photo journal" containing pictures that represent the character of New Hampshire in three categories: people, food, and nature. Students are allowed 1 hour per week of school time to work on their report. During this time, George categorizes the pictures he's taken during the previous week and pastes them into his photo album. He then writes a word or phrase about each picture. Two other students choose to organize their written report around the same categories and they often work with George during this in-school time or are invited on weekend outings with George's family when he takes some of the photographs for his report.

Step Three: Express the Overall Goal of This Lesson for all Students

If teachers are working with a familiar curriculum, one developed by others or themselves, this step should be easy and quick. For a high school English class the goal might be for students to discuss the use of dialect in two Alice Walker short stories. For a kindergarten class, the goal of a group reading activity might be for students to appreciate the rhythm of a Maurice Sendak poem. The goal of a 6th grade science lesson might be to build a small solar collector to power a low wattage light bulb. Although each of these lessons have many other secondary learning objectives, teachers need to communicate to other team members just a brief statement of the broad goal of the lesson, the materials or books that will be used, and any products that students will be required to complete during the course of the class.

Step Four: Decide How This Student Can Participate

Although the larger question for teachers is "how can I make this lesson meaningful for all my students?" teams may meet to focus on one or more students with intensive learning needs. Although there are many resources on curriculum modification available for teachers, we have developed a hierarchy of participation options that teams can use as they problem-solve upcoming lessons or activities. They incorporate three important principles: (1) multi-level instruction for students who are learning the academic content of the lesson; (2) curriculum overlapping or embedding with students focusing on objectives from the domains of communication, behavior, and/or movement; and (3) the principle of partial participation that acknowledges that all students can benefit from the lesson even if they are not completing all components of the lesson (Baumgart et al., 1982; Collicott, 1991; Giangreco, Cloninger, & Iverson, 1993).

The Student Can Participate in the Lesson or Activity Just Like Other Students

There are activities and lessons in which students with significant disabilities can participate with only minor modifications and these might include: extracurricular activities, artwork, keyboarding, music appreciation, band or chorus, listening to a story reading, or physical education and games. In these situations, the participation goals for students with disabilities are the same as those for typical students.

> Doug is on his high school's track team. He runs individually and with peers during their cool-down laps. He rides the bus to meets and warms up with the team. At home meets, Doug participates in the final race of the day, an open relay race, in which the results are not counted for league standings. Doug's coach feels it's important for Doug to run in a race, not just be the team mascot.

The Student Can Participate With Adapted Materials or Expectations

The second option is for the student to be a part of the lesson or activity, but with modifications to materials, the environment or to the teacher's expectations for the outcome. A student with limited movement of her hands could join a pottery class, in which that student's finished product is judged by a different standard than the other students. A student might be enrolled in a keyboarding class, but need a keyboard adaptation to enable the student to accurately isolate the keys. Students with writing difficulties might have the option of giving an oral report or making a video to illustrate what they have learned. In testing situations, students might be required to do fewer problems or in math they might be allowed to use a calculator to perform basic functions.

Another aspect of this category of modification is that the student can be working on a different level of academics than most of the class. For example, most students in the class might be reading 10th grade science books, while one student might use a book on the same topic obtained from the elementary school library or a publisher of high-interest, low-reading-level books. Students in a junior high school math class might be working through algebra problems, while a student with severe disabilities might be using the same materials and worksheets to work on number identification.

Michael is a 5th grader with severe cerebral palsy. Because it is difficult for him to raise his hand during class discussions, he often calls out his answer, despite a classroom rule prohibiting talking without first being called on. The usual signaling devices (bells, buzzers) were deemed too disruptive so his teacher made him a cardboard hand and attached it to the end of a ruler. Now Michael keeps his handraiser on his desk during discussion, and can easily flip it up for his teacher to see when he has a contribution to make.

Old Short-term Objective: According to a team developed behavior plan, Michael will decrease his
continued

inappropriate vocalizations during class discussions to a minimum of three times per week, with loss of recess as a consequence for noncompliance.

New Short-term Objective: Michael will use his "handraiser" to get the attention of his teacher with no more than two verbal reminders from his classmates.

Andrew takes spelling tests along with all other students in his 3rd grade class. Andrew has a different spelling test than other students, based on assessment information that shows where the gaps lie in Andrew's spelling knowledge. He has fewer words and types out the words with some physical support provided by the teaching assistant.

During his chef's class, Alex learns to prepare a checkerboard cake and a jelly roll during the dessert unit. He learns to follow a recipe (with pictures and words) to get the needed materials, to pour using a measuring cup, to mix ingredients together, to turn on the stove to a desired temperature, and to use a timer to indicate when the cooking time has ended. He is not expected to read all the directions on the recipe, but to do certain steps as directed by his cooking partners.

The Student Can Participate and Focus on Learning "Embedded Skills" in Movement, Communication, and Behavior

For some students, the goal of their participation in an activity may not include mastery of any academic content. For example, classes in social studies are rich opportunities for all students to demonstrate what they know through hands-on activities. In a 9th grade interdisciplinary unit at Souhegan High School students explored the impact of economics on environmental policy, specifically relating to the destruction of the Brazilian rainforests. All students participating in the unit were involved in constructing a table top rainforest model, also providing a student with movement and communication difficulties a wonderful opportunity to work on those skills in a fun, interactive atmosphere.

Keisha is a 2nd grader who has Rett's syndrome. Although this affects her ability to communicate and move, because of the creativity of her teacher and her peers, Keisha participates in most classroom lessons and activities. Her class is studying about ladybugs. As students finish the worksheet for the lesson, they go to Keisha to get a "good job" stamp. They assist Keisha in pressing her thumb on a red ink pad and making an oval stamp on their paper. The students then add legs, spots, and feelers to complete the ladybug stamp indicating a job well done.

Old Short-term Objective: When a brightly colored object (such as a pink cup or a red monkey) is moved across Keisha's visual field, she will move her eyes and head to track it 80% of the time for 10 consecutive trials.

New Short-term Objective: When classmates approach Keisha to talk or work on a class project that is interesting to her, she will raise her head and make eye contact with them until they leave her side and return to their desk.

Julian is a 2nd grader with severe cerebral palsy. This year he played the part of a prince in his class play. A friend taperecorded the prince's dialogue
continued

and Julian activated a switch to say his lines at the appropriate time.

Old Short-term Objective: During speech and language therapy, Julian will activate the on-off switch to play a music tape within 15 seconds of a cue on 3 out of 4 consecutive trials.

New Short-term Objective: In the context of a variety of class activities, including class performances and book reports, Julian will activate a tape loop using a switch within 10 seconds of a cue.

Matt is in an 8th grade science class, but has no traditional academic goals on his IEP. During lab experiments, he is responsible for getting his group's dissection tray organized and bringing it over to the lab station. Matt takes instant pictures of the various steps of the experiment and with the assistance of another group member, pastes them into their team's lab notebook alongside the corresponding written lab report.

Old Short-term Objective: Matt will sequence 5–6 pictures depicting a familiar activity correctly 9 times out of 10.

New Short-term Objective: During classroom activities such as science lab, Matt will improve his skills in sequencing by assembling dissection trays or by documenting the steps of the experiment by taking instant photos and pasting them in order alongside the corresponding steps of the written report.

The Student Can Be in the Classroom, But Work on an Activity That Fulfills a Different Purpose

When teams begin to consider this option they need to carefully weigh a number of factors. First, is there any way that the task can be modified to include the student with the disability? If a

student is a member of the class, but given "special work" to occupy him or her while the rest of the class does the "regular work,"
then the team needs to do additional brainstorming. Invisible barriers can be as separating and damaging as physical barriers for
students with disabilities. The team should ask, "How will it benefit the student to do different work at this time as opposed to
the same work as the rest of the class?" There might be occasions
when students with disabilities need to have a break from the
regular class routine to relax, to reduce their stress level, or to
organize their work for the next class or activity. If this is the case
and the student is doing different work for legitimate reasons, then
a proactive decision is being made. For example, typical students
may be doing math seatwork while the student with the disability is putting together a money envelope for a field trip that the
class will take later in the week. Some students may be writing
short stories while one student is listening to soothing music on
a personal tape player. If teachers structure their classroom communities for all students to have opportunities during the day for
independent work, either at their desk or at learning stations, then
this choice would not stigmatize a student with disabilities. In a
class in which students work by themselves, in pairs, or in small
groups, the student with the disability would not stand out as
different even if that student were engaged in an activity different than other students.

The decision to physically or functionally remove a student
from the core classroom activity is a serious one and needs to be
made by an entire team. It is rarely acceptable for students who
are fully included to be separated from the rest of the class, therefore it is important that the team first explore ways for the student to be involved in the lesson before utilizing this option. We
would suggest that the team involve other students in problem
solving means to include the student with disabilities. Teachers also
may wish to talk with the class about the necessity of some students doing different work some of the time.

Joe has physical disabilities that require he change
position several times during the school day. During music class he gets out of his wheelchair and
the teaching assistant or physical therapist assists
continued

him in moving his arms and legs through range-of-motion exercises. He is certainly listening to and learning from the music activities that are going on the class, but Joe's teachers have decided that scheduling this time for his exercises is the best decision, given the overall picture of Joe's day in school. Joe receives direct physical therapy from the physical therapist one day each week after school at a local hospital. This service is covered through Joe's parents' private insurance.

Mr. Mansfield lectures his science class for the first 20 minutes of each period. The students do a lab experiment or other hands-on activity for 20 minutes and then come back together to discuss their observations and results for the last 10 minutes of the period. Donald is a member of this class; he has an extremely difficult time staying with the group if the activity requires sitting or listening to the teacher talk. The team is striving to find ways for Donald to increase his ability to listen and they have enlisted some of his friends to rub his back and redirect him during lecture times. Despite trying a number of different ways to help him stay with the group, the team doesn't seem to be getting anywhere. Donald's parents are very interested in Donald having a real job when he graduates from high school and would like him to start learning a job while he is still in school. Because he likes animals, he is responsible for feeding the class guinea pig, mynah bird, and fish. He does this with the assistance of a paraprofessional during the beginning of the class lecture.

Is Leaving the Classroom Ever Acceptable for Students With Severe Disabilities?

It would be unrealistic to suggest that students with severe disablities never leave the regular education classroom during the course of the school day. Particularly for students with challenging behavior, teams must often balance the needs of typical students for a quiet learning environment with the knowledge that removing a student who is acting out provides only a short-term solution to a complicated problem. When teams are engaging in focused problem solving directed towards keeping the student in the classroom for longer and longer periods of time, we can feel more comfortable about that student leaving for brief walks or breaks. There are also situations in which students need to have personal care needs attended to that clearly need to take place outside of the classroom and that inevitably cut into instructional time.

It has been our experience that as schools become more committed to including students in regular classes, as their teachers and other staff become more competent in curriculum modification and, perhaps most importantly, when other students are fully involved in problem solving for inclusion, reliance on these latter options decreases.

Johanna is learning to express her preferences for how people help her perform basic hygiene and self-help chores. It is expected that someday she will be able to hire and supervise people who might be paid to provide those supports to her. Her physical therapist gives her the choice of where to have her therapy—in the classroom during silent reading or story time or out of the classroom in a small workroom down the hall. Some days Johanna chooses the classroom and some days she chooses to leave.

Rick is 19 and spends Mondays, Wednesdays, and Fridays at a local community college taking

continued

business courses. On Tuesdays and Thursdays he works for a company that manufacturers sterilizing equipment for hospitals and laboratories.

Leslie, a high school sophomore, works in the library second period every day. She checks books in, sorts them by color-coded binding labels, dusts credenzas, and keeps the desk area neat.

Brandon, a 9th grader, has a free period at the end of the day. A peer tutor spends time with him during this period, and, based on their joint decision, they go for a walk around the school grounds, play computer games, listen to music in the Academic Support Center, or hang out in the common areas of the 9th grade wing.

Step Five: Identify Ways That Students Can Cooperate With and Support One Another

This step was addressed in Chapter 2 in detail with examples of how students could work together during classroom lessons and other school activities.

Step Six: Plan Multi-level Lessons and Assign Responsibility for Adapting Materials or the Environment

The next step in the curriculum modification process is to decide how to teach the lesson so that all students can participate. There are eight general types of modifications or adaptations that might be implemented, which include:

1. Supplement instructions by repeating, clarifying, breaking down steps, or changing terminology. Some students may just need to have information or instructions repeated or phrased in a slightly different way for them to follow the teacher's directions. This can be done by the regular teacher as he or she moves around the room checking for students' understanding, by a peer who checks to see that cooperative teammates are following directions correctly, or by a support person who keeps an eye out for any student who appears lost.

> Erin's SLP takes advantage of art class to expand and enrich Erin's concrete and conceptual vocabulary. The SLP sits at Erin's table and while providing general assistance to all of the students, engages Erin in conversation about what she is doing, what materials she's using, which step comes next, and so on.

2. Change how instructions or information is presented. Some suggestions for targeting instructions or how information is presented include: (a) provide written or pictorial instructions for the student to refer to after oral instructions have been given to the whole class; (b) assist the student in reading written or pictorial instructions; (c) provide a demonstration that illustrates the steps in the learning activity; and (d) have a completed model to show the student—an art project, a science report, a sample math problem.

> Andrew has a difficult time understanding complex verbal instructions. His teachers have found that he learns best by copying other students or copying a model of the work that has been completed for him. When he was in kindergarten his parents fought for him to be in regular classes so that he could take advantage of learning from his peers. As he moves into 4th grade, he has learned school routines and knows his school job well because of his interest in copying his friends.

3. Change kind of output required. Students can express their knowledge in many ways. Instead of requiring the traditional written report, consider the following: videotapes or slide shows, bulletin boards, cookbooks or recipes, displays or showcases, banners, photo albums, diaries or journals, songs or other musical productions, poems, game boards, mobiles, dioramas, a speech, invention, commercial or comic strip, or model.

> Peter's social studies unit focuses on the South American countries. Groups of five students work on one country and are responsible for presenting a major project at the school's "We Are All One World" fair. Peter will learn basic Spanish phrases (greetings, common foods), make a collage of products the U.S. imports from South America, learn basic photography skills to produce a slide show of the fair, and practice cooking skills when the class sponsors a "South American Foods" bazaar.

4. Change amount or quality of output required. Requiring that the student complete fewer problems to demonstrate mastery, setting a different standard of quality (must get 50% correct instead of 100% to move on to the next set of problems), and giving a student longer to complete an assignment are examples of this modification.

> Larry is a 3rd grader who is reading at a beginning level. He enjoys participating in class activities as long as he experiences success and feels he is doing the same work as other students. The students were reviewing parts of speech by naming them on a sentence written on the blackboard. The teacher made sure to include a very simple subject-verb-object sentence and called on Larry to name the first word in the sentence for him to have success during this activity.

5. Involve students in process steps of the lesson. For almost every lesson or activity that teachers develop, there is a "doing" part of the lesson that accompanies the "thinking" part of the lesson. For some students, learning will take place primarily during the more active part of the lesson. Even lectures may have a process component. Teachers sometimes need assistance with demonstrations as they are lecturing, a student might hold a globe, use a pointer to indicate a country on a map, or hand the teacher color-coded dissection tools. Books may need to be passed out, an overhead projector might need to be set up and turned on and off, or a slide projector may need to be advanced on command from the teacher. Other students often see opportunities for involvement not noticed by teachers or specialists, so teams need to enlist students in the problem-solving process.

Many primary-age students are responsible for morning milk routine. To make the routine a rich learning opportunity for all students, some teachers structure the task the following way. Photographs of all the children are mounted on 3" × 3" heavy cardboard, labeled with first names and laminated. These are kept in alphabetical order in a small file box. When students arrive in the morning, they find their picture and put it in the "white milk" basket or the "red milk" basket. A few minutes before snack time, two students (including one student with a disability) count the number of pictures in each basket and go to the cafeteria to pick up the corresponding number of "white" (regular) and "red" (low-fat) milk containers. If the student with the disability knows classmates by name, the child hands containers to classmates with direction from a buddy ("Kevin, give this one to Shawna. Give this one to Raphael.") If the student doesn't know students by name a child can look at each picture and find the classmate. Another option would be for students to file past the milk crates and pick up whichever kind of milk they ordered. At the end of the day, students take turns returning the pictures to the file box in alphabetical order.

---

6. Make an adaptation to the environment or provide an assistive device. Although technology isn't the total answer to including students with disabilities in regular classes, there are high-tech and low-tech adaptations that can make their participation easier. Among these are: braille books or books on tape; augmentative communication devices; high-interest picture books; adaptive switches for household machines such as blenders, tape recorders and VCRs; commercially available synopses of literature books; seating adaptations to help students work at the same height as others; adapted computer keyboards; and a variety of homemade adaptations that a weekend handyperson could build with guidance from OTs or physical therapists (PTs).

Johanna is a 2nd grader with multiple disabilities. She has a long attention span and loves watching other children act out plays or tell stories. Each child in Johanna's class must do a report on an endangered animal. Johanna's friends help her narrow down her choices by asking her to pick her "favorite animal" by eye gazing at pictures of animals on the covers of nature magazines. She chooses the panda. Johanna's assistant asks a small group of Johanna's peers to name "words that Johanna will need to use if she writes a story about pandas." The assistant then makes a series of overlays using panda-related vocabulary words—black, white, big, bamboo, China, cubs. Responding to "yes and no" questions and eye gazing to indicate her choice of words, Johanna communicates what she wants to write about. Her assistant turns Johanna's one-word responses into narrative, reads it back to Johanna for confirmation and has Johanna illustrate a cover for the report using an ink pad and stamp set. A classmate might read Johanna's story aloud during sharing time or Johanna could activate a tape-recorded version of a classmate reading her story.

---

7. Provide physical assistance. At times, just the provision of simple physical assistance enables students with disabilities to participate in ways more nearly like their peers. Facilitated communication requires minimal physical assistance to enable some students with severe communication and/or motor difficulties (e.g. autism, cerebral palsy) to communicate and do academic work using a computer or Canon Communicator. Peers can help their classmate by learning how to facilitate. Other examples of physical assistance include involving friends to assist with warm-up exercises in gym, providing hand-over-hand assistance in labs or home economics, and providing sighted guidance to students who are blind. Being provided with such assistance may mean the difference between sitting on the sidelines or joining in with classmates.

> Brian is a 5th grader who loves music and can keep time with his hands and feet beautifully. He had difficulty following the dance directions called out by the P.E. teacher when they did a folk dance unit. Brian's classmates eagerly volunteered to be his partner and guide him through the dance patterns. During the dances he sits out, Brian and his peers provide percussion through clapping and foot stomping.
>
> *Old Short-term Objective:* During physical education activities for which he is unable to participate, Brian will be provided alternative activities by the adapted physical education teacher.
>
> *New Short-term Objective:* With adaptations or modifications, Brian will participate with peer assistance in all physical education, art, and music classes.

> Alex, a 10th grader with significant disabilities, uses his a laptop computer to do work in his English literature class. When he wants to answer a question or offer an opinion, he uses an alphabet board and when he sees his friends in the hall, a high-five is the only system he needs.

8. Help the student do part of the task. It is better for students with disabilities to be in regular classes doing only part of what their friends are doing than to be in segregated classrooms completing nonfunctional tasks (Baumgart et al., 1982).

> Although Michael has severe cerebral palsy and will always have difficulty writing legibly, he is required to print some of his written work each day because the OT feels that it is very good exercise for his hands. Michael types final copies of his written work using a keyboard adaptation on his word processor.

Step Seven: Continue to Problem-Solve Participation Through Systematic Observation of Regular Class Lessons and Other Integrated Activities

Students with severe disabilities benefit from being members of regular classes—they learn important skills, establish friendships with typical students, and generally enjoy being a part of the unpredictable regular world. The planning process presented here has relied on classroom teachers, parents, and specialists working together to plan activities and to decide ahead of time how to best involve the student with disabilities. To truly include students with disabilities requires a full repertoire of participation ideas and strategies; curriculum modification, evaluation, and problem solving must be ongoing. Teams need to meet on a regular basis—for some students once a week, for others a bit less often—to talk about how things went during a previous week and to make plans for instruction during the coming week. Team members also need to be able to adapt to unexpected changes in the classroom schedule and format.

All teams have their own personalities. Some are very organized and thrive in orderly team meetings, others are looser and come up with their best ideas during conversations while on playground duty. To suggest that all teams use one planning process defies what we know about communication and collaboration. Regardless of a given team's style, the following structured process for observing in regular classes can help teams in finding better ways to include the student with disabilities. As presented in Chapter 2, this process and the recording form (see Figure 3–1) were utilized by Josh's team to gather information about Josh's inclusion in 5th grade.

Gathering comprehensive information about how the student with disabilities is functioning in the regular class can enable teams to improve the quality and level of participation. This observation process is particularly useful for teams working with students who have challenging behaviors; these teams need detailed information about how the student behaves in a variety of environments, during different activities, and when interacting with different people.

The following steps will be helpful in conducting classroom observations. Sample questions are included that help the team to consider the variables in the class.

Step 1. On a rotating basis, team members should observe the regular class in which the student is included. The observer should take notes on what the teacher and other students are doing, what the targeted student is doing, and who is providing support to the student. Team members who do observations on a regular basis

FUNCTIONAL ANALYSIS OF OPPORTUNITIES TO PARTICIPATE IN REGULAR SCHOOL ACTIVITIES

Student: _____   School/Grade: _____

Class/Activity: _____   Observation Date: _____

Physical/Social Setting: _____

OBSERVATION DATA		Recorder: _____	
Time	Class/Activity	What is student doing?	Support

FIGURE 3–1
Regular Classroom Observation Recording Form

report they "see more" when they are observing than when they are providing instruction or other support to the student. Table 3–2 displays a menu of questions that can help focus the observer's note taking.

Shayne, a 1st grader with significant disabilities, has surpassed everyone's expectations by gaining some preliteracy skills. Although he can't read or write whole words yet, the creative adaptation of worksheets and lessons allow him to be involved in all language arts activities. One week his reading group worked on the story "The Queen's Hat." Shayne's activities included circling all of the hats on a photocopy of the book, circling all of the "hat" words by matching to a "hat" sample, coloring a big picture of a hat, making a hat out of newspaper, using a highlighter and marking all the letter "H"s in the story, counting the hats, retelling the main points of the story into a tape recorder, and copying some of the characters' names from a sample.

Step 2. Make copies of the observation forms and bring them to the next team meeting. Before the team discussion, each team member should review the observations and note preliminary ideas for increasing the student's participation.

Erin, who has Down syndrome, participated in her school's field day. Although she has no serious physical limitations, Erin has been reluctant to participate in new activities. She is afraid of taking risks, of falling down, or of failing. As Erin's mother observed from the sidelines with the other parents, she remarked on her daughter's willingness to participate. As Erin handed her mother her glasses before climbing up on the trampoline, her mother
continued

TABLE 3–2
Questions to guide regular class observations

What is the general setup of the room? Dividers? Learning centers? Lab tables? Sewing stations? Cooking stations?

Can all students use desks, materials, equipment? How are the students' desks arranged?

Is the lighting consistent in different parts of the room? Is the room warm, cold?

Does the teacher use audiovisual equipment? Does the teacher write on the chalkboard? Legibly? Easy to see from all seats?

What materials are used during the lesson? Do students have the materials in their desks? Do students pass out materials to other students? Are students required to get supplies from a central location in the classroom?

How long does it take for students to prepare for the beginning of the lesson once the period begins?

How much student interaction is required/allowed during the lesson? Is it necessary for students to move around the room to accomplish the goals of the lesson?

What is the teacher saying and doing? How much of the class is lecture versus group work versus individual seatwork? What does the teacher do when students are engaged in individual seatwork or small group activities?

What is the noise level in the class?

How do students seek help from the teacher? Do students freely ask for and receive help from other students?

How does the teacher present tasks? Does the teacher lecture? Does the teacher frequently call on students to verify that they understand the material? Does the teacher ask questions that show understanding? Memorization of facts? Analysis? Contrast and comparison?

How does the teacher monitor students' progress during the course of the period? How does the teacher provide feedback to students? How often? Positive or negative?

How does the teacher maintain order in the classroom?

If there are other adults in the classroom what is their role? Which students do they help?

How do students know that the period/lesson is over?

exclaimed "I never expected her to try this one . . . she's always been too afraid of falling down. I'm really surprised!"

Old Short-term Objective: Erin will meet with the school guidance counselor to discuss appropriate ways to make friends, one 20-minute session one time per week for the spring semester.

New Short-term Objective: Each week, Erin will invite one friend to her house for an after-school or weekend activity.

Step 3. At the next team meeting, discuss which classes or times of the day present significant challenges. Using the observation notes, team members should explore how the student's participation could be enhanced, how the activity could be revised to better include the student, how other students might be utilized to provide more natural supports, and finally, determine if the student's priority learning objectives are being addressed in the class.

Step 4. Distribute a summary of the meeting and copies of the observation forms to team members not present. Expanding the team meeting report to include these items is done not to generate more paper, but rather to enable the team to look at both "the forest and the trees." In assessing the student's involvement in the regular class it is important to document what is working and to fix what isn't in a timely fashion.

Lisa is a 7th grader. Her parents' number one goal is to have their daughter increase her levels of cooperation and participation with peers both in academic and social settings. In science class, members of her group help her hold and manipulate various objects during experiments. During music, Lisa sits next to friends who help her sway to the beat of the music. During home economics, Lisa assists with stirring, mixing, and shaping of dough and cookie mix. In language arts, Lisa enjoys listening to poetry being read by her friends. And during art class she is learning to work with different art media such as clay, paper mache, and finger paint.

Old Short-term Objective: With verbal prompting from her aide, Lisa will demonstrate cause and effect by pressing a switch that activates a toy on the busy box (e.g., the monkey that plays cymbals) 3 out of 4 times for 20 consecutive trials.

New Short-term Objective: With partial physical assistance of a peer and when she is feeling well, Lisa will reach out toward materials and objects she enjoys, such as art materials, books, and musical instruments. Achievement of objective will be measured by peer and teacher interviews.

◼️ PLANNING AND RECORDING IEP OBJECTIVES AND GENERAL CLASS PARTICIPATION

In Chapter 2, a matrix form was utilized by Josh's team to record some "informed guesses" for how his priority learning objectives would be addressed in the 5th grade class and other school environments. Because Josh had not yet been included in the class, the team could only express Josh's learning in very general terms. For example, for the objective "make choices" the team thought that he might learn that skill by choosing books during language arts, by choosing who to sit next to at snack time, and to select an activity when the teacher set up exploratory stations in science.

After Josh had been in school for about a month and various team members had the opportunity to observe him in a variety of lessons and school activities, they conducted baseline assessment of certain skills, based on his family's priorities. (Table 3–3 presents Josh's priority annual goals again.)

From this information, the team was able to write short-term objectives that projected their best estimate of how Josh's skills would change over the course of the year. They recognized that their projections would need to be modified based on the changes in Josh that would occur and the effectiveness of instruction, so they left open the possibility of revising the objectives frequently,

TABLE 3–3
Josh's annual IEP goals

1. Within real-life situations, such as choosing food in the lunchroom, selecting books in the library, or picking friends to be on his team in gym, Josh will make a choice from among five choices in each category.
2. When talking with a responsive peer, Josh will take three conversational turns using his communication book or natural gestures.
3. When doing errands, on trips to the boys rooms, or at other times, Josh will independently walk to familiar rooms within the school building.
4. Josh will demonstrate an understanding of one-to-one correspondence by passing out materials such as books, milk cartons, or art supplies to peers in class.
5. The making friends priority was not included on Josh's IEP as a behavioral goal for him, but was rather addressed through the development of a circle of friends.
6. During arrival and dismissal times, Josh will independently manage the belongings in his knapsack.
7. The interacting with friends priority was not written as an IEP goal but was addressed by staff and family working to get Josh enrolled in the after-school latch-key program and one town recreation department sport each semester.
8. In cooperation with a peer, Josh will work in the school's recycling program 3 days per week.

rather than using them as static benchmarks of progress to be evaluated at artificial times throughout the year (report card or progress report time).

Josh's team realized that he would be learning a great deal more than what was specified on his IEP, and they wanted a record of how he was taking advantage of the rich, regular class environment. They met on a weekly basis to discuss upcoming units, lessons, and activities, and to decide how Josh would participate in them. Using the curriculum modification strategies described in the first part of this chapter, they were able to brainstorm lots of ways for him to be involved. Some of his participation was anticipated during these planning sessions, but to be honest, the classroom teacher, other students, and support staff had to be constantly on the lookout for opportunities for Josh to participate, and needed to be flexible and creative to help him take advantage of those opportunities.

One subject area that seemed to be particularly challenging for the team was science class. The beginning of the year observation showed Josh sitting a lot during class and involved mostly as a "gofer" for materials and supplies. During one of the first weekly planning sessions involving the whole team, they decided to focus on science as the priority for their creative planning efforts.

Many teams have found it useful to use a form like that presented in Figure 3–2 (Regular Class Instructional Planning Form) to structure their discussion of how students would participate in future lessons. The classroom teacher, a related service provider, or an inclusion facilitator could take notes during the planning meeting and then make copies for all team members and Josh's file.

The classroom teacher described the overall goal of a given lesson, the materials that would be used, how students would be grouped, and what homework assignments, projects, and tests would be used to evaluate students' learning. The team then discussed, "how Josh will be involved." In this case, the week-long unit was on astronomy. Both science and language arts time would be utilized every day to emphasize the integration of certain language arts skills (library skills, outlining, factual writing, speaking in front of a group), cooperative skills (assigning responsibilities among team members, cooperating during a group presentation), and science concepts (learning about constellations and one planet in the solar system). Every day, the teacher would present some lecture information for about 15–20 minutes that the students had to record in their notebooks. Students would be allowed to go to the library in teams to obtain reference materials on their chosen planet, and they would be given any remaining class time to write their section of the report, make posters or drawings of their planet, or rehearse their group presentation. The team reviewed Josh's IEP objectives and decided that during most of the unit, Josh would be working on embedded skills in the areas of movement and communication, but that his participation in the group was an important learning outcome that was not represented on his IEP.

The team's ideas were recorded on the form and it became part of Josh's 5th grade folder, along with samples of his work accumulated throughout the year. The last column is for team members to keep a running record of Josh's progress.

Student: _Josh Brooks_

Description of Lesson/Unit: _Astronomy: Constellations and Planets_

What Will the Class Be Doing?	Materials/Homework/Tests/Projects	How Can Student Participate	IEP Objectives Being Addressed	Support Needed
Learning and mapping constellations	Dial-A-Constellation wheels	Connect dots/stars on constellation map	Make choices	Remind students in Josh's group about using his communication system and giving him a role
Listening to some lecture material	Library books and posters	Look at books	Sustain interactions	SLP will be in class M & F
Going to library in small groups	Paper and pencil test at end of unit - recognize constellations, characteristics of nine planets	Distinguish between planets	Make friends	OT will work with Josh's group on Wednesday
Reading about astronomy	Paper mache'	Make model of planet with paper mache'		Teaching assistant will be in class for part of period on T & Th
Group presentation - maybe posters, models	Posterboard Paints	Color poster		Josh will be in Mr. Rounds' group at Planatarium
Writing individual sections of report		Illustrate cover of report/folder		
Visiting planatarium next week - Tues a.m.		*Remember to get bus with seat belts for field trip		

FIGURE 3-2
Instructional Planning Matrix

■ SUMMARY

This chapter concludes the first section of the book. In Chapter 1, a chronological presentation of best practices in special education was presented. Current best practices for students with severe disabilities suggest that full inclusion results in better social and educational outcomes. In Chapter 2, a comprehensive process was described for building the foundation for a student's education program. That foundation includes getting to know the student by focusing on personality, talents and needs rather than on deficits; identifying the student's priority educational goals for the upcoming year; and, brainstorming creative ideas and supports which enable the student to fully participate in an age-appropriate regular classroom. In Chapter 3, specific inclusive classroom examples are presented which illustrate the principles that underlie the development and personalization of curriculum for all students in the classroom.

Chapters 4 and 5 focus the task of instructional planning on ways that communication technology, support, and instruction can enhance participation and learning. Alternatives to traditional "communication assessment and programming" are presented, highlighting a new role for speech-language pathologists in relation to other team members.

■ REFERENCES

Baumgart, D., Brown, L., Pumpian, I., Nisbet, J., Ford, A., Sweet, M., Messina, R., & Schroeder, J. (1982). Principle of partial participation and individualized adaptations in educational programs for severely handicapped students. *Journal of the Association for the Severely Handicapped, 7,* 17–27.

Collicott, J. (1991). Implementing multi-level instruction: Strategies for classroom teachers. In G. Porter & D. Richler (Eds.), *Changing Canadian schools: Perspectives on disability and inclusion* (pp. 191–218). North York, Ontario: G. Allan Roeher Institute.

Ford, A., Davern, L., Meyer, L., Schnorr, R., Black, J., & Dempsey, P. (1989). Overview. In A. Ford, B. Schnorr, L. Meyer, L. Davern, J. Black, & P. Dempsey (Eds.), *The Syracuse community-referenced curriculum guide for students with moderate and severe disabilities* (pp. 3–13). Baltimore: Paul H. Brookes Publishing Co.

Giangreco, M., Cloninger, C., & Iverson, V. (1993). *Choosing options and accommodations for children (COACH): A guide to planning inclusive education.* Baltimore: Paul H. Brookes Publishing Co.

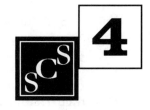

Designing and Implementing Communicative Assessments in Inclusive Settings

Stephen N. Calculator

■❑ INTRODUCTION

The preface and first three chapters of this book have aquainted readers with a variety of strategies for supporting students with severe disabilities in inclusive classrooms. As we noted in Chapter 1, best practices that evolved in education (e.g., the use of more environmentally referenced assessments, movement towards transdisciplinary models of service delivery, increased involvement of families and classmates, focus on enhanced levels of participation) quickly began to influence practices in the area of communication as well. As settings for instruction moved to regular classrooms, it became imperative to identify learning needs and to measure learning outcomes relative to expectations in general education. Chapter 2 described strategies for getting to know students and methods of identifying students' instructional priorities. In Chapter 3, readers were encouraged to examine communication in the broader contexts of inclusion and participation.

The present chapter will build on these earlier themes, operating on the premise that communication assessments must be conceived and implemented in the context of general education curricula. This chapter begins with an anecdote to illustrate *negative consequences* that may arise when team members introduce their own individual curricula (in assessment) rather than proceeding from a shared perspective. Best practices for conducting communication assessments are reviewed, with corresponding examples. Next, a series of case studies drawn from actual consultations by the author (SC) are presented. These reports illustrate strategies discussed elsewhere in the chapter. Finally, a self-assessment exercise is provided for readers to examine their recognition of best practices.

Teams Function Best When Playing on the Same Field

Two years ago, I was asked to provide assistance to a school district that had recently begun including students with severe disabilities in regular classrooms. Staff were seeking specific, objective feedback from an "outsider" about the quality of their special education programs. The school was transitioning from a model of service delivery that was almost exclusively pull-out, to one in which the majority of students' special needs (speech-language, occupational therapy [OT], physical therapy [PT], and so forth) were now being addressed in classrooms and related settings.

In the course of my appraisal, I had the opportunity to participate in a particularly memorable meeting of an evaluation team. This was a team of highly competent professionals who were struggling to find linkages between their professional expertise and a student's (Phil's) instructional needs.

Like other teams, these professionals grappled with inconsistencies between their respective assessment findings, and classroom teachers' observations and impressions of Phil. In the course of this meeting, team members identified a need to adapt a perspective (concerning Phil) that transcended the boundaries of their respective disciplines. They determined that each team member's assessment results were only valid and useful to the extent that they clarified the nature of Phil's abilities and needs, and outlined corresponding strategies by which these same factors could be addressed in different instructional settings. In other words, team members supported the need for a common field of play on which to pursue their respective tasks.

Phil had suffered a severe head trauma 3 years earlier. He continued to display a variety of behavioral and language/learning disabilities, such as difficulty maintaining attention, verbal perseverations, and frequent off-topic responses. Phil's 4th grade classroom teacher and aide were unusually adept in working together to modify tasks and expectations of him. As a result, he was successfully participating in a modified curriculum, performing at and even above grade level in some subject areas.

In preparation for developing his individualized educational plan (IEP) for the next school year, the evalution team convened to update Phil's progress. The OT began the meeting by discussing the results of her formal testing. She reported that Phil's coordination and balance had improved significantly since he had been enrolled in her program. Each day, Phil was required to walk across a beam during physical education class. The OT suggested that this program might be suspended next year in light of Phil's progress.

As she spoke, I recalled seeing Phil attempt to pull his boots on prior to going out for recess the day before. Phil stood in the middle of the room, brought one foot up, and lurched several feet to one side. Subsequent attempts netted the same results. Next, he brought his boot to his teacher, asking for assistance. Phil was encouraged to do it himself. Phil then positioned himself in a corner, with his back against the two walls, and finally pulled on his boots. Although Phil was able to walk across a beam in gym class, his lack of balance caused him
continued

difficulty getting dressed and maneuvering around the classroom.

The OT then reported the results of visual-motor testing. Once again, Phil's scores on tests requiring him to match and copy geometric designs, draw a line through a maze, and so forth were significantly improved since previous testing. Again, I recalled an interview with Phil's teacher in which she reported that Phil was often frustrated by his inability to copy information from the blackboard.

Next, the SLP presented the results of her testing. The team was suddenly confronted with a barage of age equivalents, grade equivalents, z scores, t scores, stanines, and percentiles. The report concluded with the SLP profiling Phil's strengths and weaknesses across the various dimensions of language.

While I concurred with her findings, I found myself wondering whether the SLP had overlooked some of Phil's more significant problems. Again, while observing Phil in his classroom, I noted several problems that appeared to hinder the quality of his interactions with others. These were shared at the time with Phil's teacher, for confirmation. His teacher raised additional concerns about Phil's communication, then prioritized *our* observations relative to the extent that each behavior appeared to limit Phil's participation in class.

Several behaviors were cited as top priorities:

1. Phil often had problems realizing when to stop talking. In responding to questions, he often continued to drone on and on, providing information that was often irrelevant, redundant, and/or of little interest to classmates. The teacher found herself fighting the impulse to avoid calling on Phil. Classmates exchanged pained expressions with one another each time Phil was called on in class. Other students rarely asked Phil for assistance, despite his strong abilities in certain academic areas. They were frustrated when their questions went unanswered, or Phil responded off-topic.

2. Teachers and other staff were often annoyed by Phil's tendency to blurt out inappropriate comments during class. For example, in the middle of a teacher's lecture, or during silent reading, Phil might exclaim, "That's really stupid!" They attributed these behaviors to Phil's problems inhibiting such remarks.

3. Phil was regarded by some teachers and students as disrespectful. He often interrupted others, rather than waiting for his turn to speak. When addressed, he often looked away from the speaker and began working independently. Again, these behaviors annoyed others.

Returning to the team meeting, we then heard from the resource room specialist. Achievement test results were recounted, and the team was subjected to another string of stanines, z scores, and percentiles. The specialist called attention to the *facts* that math and reading comprehension continued to be particularly weak areas for Phil.

At this stage of the meeting, I noticed that Phil's classroom teacher appeared to be losing interest in the proceedings. She shifted her glance from her watch to the window and to the door. The rest of the team appeared to share this teacher's lack of enthusiasm for what had been transpiring at the meeting.

Unable to remain a passive observer any longer, I turned to the classroom teacher and asked, "How is Phil doing in math?" She replied that it was a strong area for Phil. In fact, she was often pressed to find tasks that challenged him sufficiently, and were still pertinent to other class members. Another team member asked about Phil's reading abilities. His teacher reported that Phil's comprehension was largely dependent on whether the reading material was selected by herself or by Phil, the amount of time he had to process the material, the degree to which the material engaged his interest, and his

continued

health status. However, she once again reported that reading was not an area of concern.

At this time, Phil's case manager encouraged team members to reflect on how the meeting had progressed to that point. All reported feelings that these meetings were largely a waste of time, as were the hours of testing which preceded them. Phil's teacher indicated that she dreaded these meetings and resented being removed from her classroom only to be bombarded with information that never seemed to be useful in meeting her students' needs.

Like other teachers whom I had interviewed previously (and since), Phil's teacher was unable to recall, much less explain, his IEP goals and objectives. Most teachers I have spoken to report that they have not reviewed their students' goals for months and, in some cases, are unable to even locate these plans. This is in stark contrast to the notion of IEPs as "living documents."

Phil's team resolved that in the future they would make greater attempts to supplement formal testing and other discipline-specific procedures with classroom observations, teacher interviews, and examination of students' work (e.g., portfolio review). This would result in different team members designing and interpreting assessment results based on similar sources of information. Phil's teachers and parents were not looking for SLP, OT, PT, and LD recommendations. Instead, they sought methods of enhancing Phil's participation at school (and elsewhere) through improvements in communication, visual-motor, gross motor, social, and other abilities.

This section began by proposing that effective team functioning requires team members to step out on fields of play that may vary from the ones for which they were trained professionally, yet resemble the arenas that other profesessionals and parents encounter daily. Throughout this book, communication is examined as a means of fostering students' interaction and participation in inclusive settings.

We propose inclusion as an organizing construct through which all assessment activities are conducted, irrespective of whether our primary purpose(s) are to: (1) determine students' eligibility for communication services; (2) determine students' present levels of ability; (3) identify instructional goals and objectives; or (4) evaluate the effectiveness of instruction (Noonan & Siegel-Causey, 1990; Richard & Schiefelbusch, 1990). In the following sections of this chapter, principles and procedures that are consistent with the first three of these purposes are described. Chapter 5 provides a comprehensive discussion of methods for evaluating the effectiveness of communication instruction, and the degree to which such instruction promotes inclusion (Table 5–3).

Determining A Student's Eligibility for Communication Services

Suggested considerations for determining students who are candidates for communication services are summarized in Table 4–1. SLPs (with input from other team members) are often asked to identify and prioritize students who need communicative instruction. They may also be asked for their opinions about whether direct or indirect (e.g., consultative) speech-language services are warranted for students. It is important to maintain a distinction here: Students may be identified as having communication needs and yet be determined low priorities for contact with the SLP. Communication should none the less pervade students' curricula, with or without direct involvement from SLPs.

Phrased somewhat differently, the fact that direct contact with an SLP is not recommended (by the team) should not preclude a student from receiving communication instruction. It only indicates that the student's communication needs can be addressed through other means, as would be the case for classmates without disabilities. In many of these cases, informal contact is maintained with the SLP, who continues to monitor students' progress and changing status.

TABLE 4–1
Bases for determining students' eligibility for communication services

1. A student who is viewed as a poor candidate for intervention with an SLP may still be viewed as a high priority for communicative instruction.
2. **All** students can benefit from communicative interventions that foster interaction and participation in different settings.
3. There are no minimal criteria, or prerequisites, that must be in place to justify communication services.
4. Eligibility for speech-language services should be the prerogative of a qualified/certified SLP (with team consensus), whose decision considers each student's individual needs. (ASHA, 1989)
5. Discrepancies across language areas, or between language and related skills (e.g., intellectual functioning) can be useful in predicting students' abilities to benefit from services, to the extent that such measures are valid.
6. Eligibility decisions must consider existing environmental demands for communication that are being placed on students, and students' abilities (or potential, with instruction) to meet these demands.
7. Eligibility decisions must also anticipate future communication demands and opportunites, beyond school.

Zero Exclusion

We believe very strongly that **all** students can benefit from communication intervention that focuses on fostering and enhancing interaction and participation in different settings. There are no minimal criteria or prerequisites that must be in place to justify communication services.

Unfortunately, this philosophy contradicts current practices in many places. Casby (1992) reported that 31 of the 50 states in the United States use discrepancy formula (examining communication skills relative to cognitive functioning) to identify students who are eligible for communication services. Some criteria specify minimum standards for eligibility (e.g., services are not provided for students whose cognitive abilities fail to exceed Piaget's sensorimotor stage IV). They operate under the premise that communication instruction should not be provided until students are ready and able to benefit from it.

To the contrary, we support a position that all students communicate from birth on, irrespective of their cognitive abilities. Some students may communicate more conventionally than others, some may be more effective communicators than others, different students rely on different modes of communication, but all students communicate. Irrespective of their cognitive abilities, communication demands persist throughout the day, as do students' responses to these demands, ready or not.

Discrepancy Formulas

Other criteria (for eligibility) stress discrepancies between one or more areas of communication (phonology, syntax, semantics, and pragmatics) and intellectual functioning. Here, communication services may only be deemed necessary for students whose mental ages (as measured by **nonverbal** tests of intelligence) significantly exceed their communicative abilities. Objective criteria are offered (e.g., overall language delay of 2 or more years below mental age; language abilities falling 1.5 SD or more below the mean [for their mental age]; performance below a given percentile [for their mental age]). This suggests "room for growth" of communication skills, to the extent that cognitive measures set prognostic ceilings for expected levels of communicative skills.

These discrepancy criteria operate under the misconception that students can only progress (in communication) to a level commensurate with their mental age. To the contrary, students may demonstrate communication skills beyond that predicted by their mental age (Miller, Chapman, & Bedrosian, 1977). There is also evidence that students, whose language abilities are already commensurate with cognitive ability, derive as much benefit from language instruction as those who exhibit discrepancies between these developmental domains (Cole, Dale, & Mills,1990).

While discrepancy formula use objective criteria, such criteria often fail to predict the impact of a communication problem on a particular student. In addition, scores used to make these decisions are often based (primarily, if not exclusively) on formal tests which, themselves, are often invalid for many of these students. Readers are referred to American Speech and Hearing Association (ASHA) (1989) for further discussion regarding the misuse of discrepancy formula in identifying students with communication problems.

An Alternative to Discrepancy Formula

The ASHA (1989) subcommittee concluded that determining eligibility for speech-language services should be the prerogative of a qualified/certified SLP, whose decision considers each student's individual needs. We would elaborate here to suggest that any decisions concerning students' needs, and program options, must be based on team consensus.

Discrepancies across different developmental domains (language and cognition) or between different aspects of communication (production and comprehension) can be useful in predicting students' abilities to benefit from communication instruction. For example, a student who functions cognitively in the profound range of mental retardation may have fewer options (in terms of possible communication systems, methods of depicting symbols, ease and rate of learning, and so forth) than one who is less challenged intellectually.

It is important to remember, however, that the usefulness of discrepancy (and any other) data hinges on the validity of tests and other procedures from which they are derived. Leary and Boscardin (1992) issued four recommendations when assessing students with severe disabilities: (1) Use tests that are normed on a representative population (to our knowledge, there are no standardized tests of communication for this heterogeneous population); (2) Shift the emphasis from formal tests to curriculum-based, criterion-referenced measures; (3) In moving towards criterion-referenced tests, assess students' abilities to benefit from instruction, in the context of their modified curriculum; and (4) Supplement examiner's observations, and test results, with reports from teachers, parents and others. (Note: These recommendations are reflected in the procedures described throughout this chapter and are thus not discussed further at this time.).

We, too, suggest that formal discrepancy data must be accompanied by information about students' communicative abilities relative to present *and anticipated* demands in inclusive environments. The transition from school to work (the subject of Chapter 6) should engender major changes in communication demands, expectations, and, we hope, opportunities for our students.

Determining a Student's Present Level(s) of Communicative Ability

In addition to determining students' eligibility for communication services from SLPs and others, a second purpose of assessment might be to evaluate students' present levels of communicative ability (Noonan & Siegel-Causey,1990; Richard & Schiefelbusch, 1990). The SLP (and others) may be particularly interested in determining: (1) how a student communicates; (2) the purposes and communicative intents of students' messages; and (3) whether a student's communicative behavior is intentional.

Determining How a Student Communicates

As discussed earlier in this chapter, we contend that **all** students communicate, yet the effectiveness with which they do so varies in different settings and with different partners. A student may fail to exhibit communication skills in one setting, despite displaying these same skills in another. Thus, it is essential that communication assessments incorporate data from a variety of contexts. The case of Donald illustrates this point.

Donald was in a self-contained classroom in which all of the students communicated through nonconventional and highly ambiguous means. The students relied heavily on their teacher and other staff to assign meaning to their communicative attempts. When students attempted to communicate with one another, they were usually ignored. Probably acknowledging this, they directed the vast majority of their messages to their teacher.

Donald also attended a public school 6th grade classroom two afternoons each week. Assessments of Donald in his self-contained and regular classrooms revealed vastly different inventories and levels of communicative skill. The regular classroom offered multiple opportunities for communication with a wide range of people. Here, Donald initiated requests to peers, responded to peers' requests (e.g., gave objects on request), exchanged greetings, requested attention from his teacher and classmates, and so forth. The fact that many of these behaviors were not observed in the self-contained classroom

continued

---

was more an artifact of this setting than a lack of skill (or consistency) on Donald's part.

Staff agreed that it would be inappropriate to attempt to enhance Donald's communication in the self-contained program, since skills that might be targeted were already in Donald's repertoire. Instead, Donald was integrated into a regular classroom, where communication goals and appropriate supports were implemented and changes in communicative functioning monitored.

Communication: It's More Than Just a Lot of Talk

It has been our experience that teachers, parents, and others often use the terms "speech" and "communication" synonymously. This often results in communication referrals that first indicate that a student has no present means of communication, and then go on to summarize different behaviors the student is exhibiting to exert control over the environment. These latter behaviors may not have previously been identified nor responded to by listeners as communicative attempts, and thus resulted in the specific negative consequences that precipitated the referral. This was certainly the case with Shelley, a 6-year-old student.

By the time I had the opportunity to observe Shelley, she had already alienated the majority of her classmates and teachers. When I asked them about Shelley's present means of communication, I was told, "She does not communicate." Staff grew increasingly impatient as I continued my interview, inquiring about Shelley's ways of communicating wants and needs, feelings, and so forth. Finally, I was told that Shelley had no means of communicating and that was why they had requested my assistance. They wanted *me* to provide her with a method of communication.

In the first 5 minutes of my observation of Shelley, I saw her aide offer three different toys. It quickly became clear that Shelley was quite communicative, but not so with the people with whom she was interacting. (Note: material in parentheses represents the examiner's impressions of Shelley's intended meanings.) Each time, Shelley ignored her aide's offer, making no attempt to reach towards the object. ("I don't want that"/reject). With the aide's verbal prodding, she then briefly glanced at a toy, picked it up for a moment, and then tossed it over her right shoulder to the floor ("Don't give me that"/refusal; "I don't want it"/rejection). Finally, her aide selected a toy that interested Shelley. This time, Shelley reached for the toy ("I want that"/request). She held it close to her body ("I like this"/comment, or, sharing feelings).

After a minute or so, I asked the aide to take this preferred toy away. Shelley reacted by clutching the toy tightly and screaming ("Stop it. Leave me alone"/protest). The aide withdrew. Several minutes later, Shelley dropped the toy on her lap tray ("I'm all done with this"/cessation).

At this point, I shared my initial impressions about Shelley's means of communication with her aide and teachers. Their help was recruited as play reconvened and, *together*, we continued identifying Shelley's means of communication.

Shelley's subsequent communication program emphasized:

1. Making certain that her classmates and teachers understood that Shelley's behavior was communicative.
2. Encouraging others to respond appropriately and contingently to Shelley's communicative attempts.
3. Encouraging teachers and classmates to model more effective (efficient, less ambiguous, socially appropriate) methods of communication for Shelley.

4. Developing an AAC system (gestures and pictures) that provided a clear means for Shelley to express messages in the contexts in which they were necessary.

Purposes and Intents of Messages

We have found Donnellan, Mirenda, Mesaros, and Fassbender's (1984) observational tool (Figure 4–1) to be useful in ascertaining how students communicate, and for what purposes. Their protocol is especially helpful in delineating the means (horizontal axis) and communicative functions (vertical axis) of challenging behaviors such as Shelley's throwing objects and screaming. We have used this tool in staff training to broaden others' perceptions of what constitutes communication behavior. Here, we stress the dual importance of fostering students' use of more conventional, socially acceptable modes of communication (left to right progression on the horizontal axis), through which they can convey a full range of communicative intents.

Once a student's present means of communication are identified, decisions are made (by the team) about the need to introduce augmentative and alternative communication (AAC) systems. As indicated earlier, AAC options are considered when the team determines that the student's present communication system is insufficient for fostering interactions and participation in inclusive settings. For example, while Shelley had various means of communication at her disposal, they were highly ambiguous, often unsuccessful, and frequently resulted in others' excluding her from activities. The team determined it was in her interest, and within her capabilities, to learn other ways of conveying different intents.

Reichle, Feeley, and Johnston (1993) identified several circumstances under which it may be necessary to change students' existing methods of communication. These considerations, summarized in Table 4–2, respect the fact that while all behavior has communicative value, there are occasions when some methods of communication are less preferable than others. Examples are presented below.

Reasons for Modifying a Student's Communicative Behavior

The behavior is socially unacceptable. This determination requires input from parents, teachers, classmates, and others. Students with severe disabilities may be ostracized when they live by cultural norms that depart significantly from those valued by their classmates. For example, while we may think it would be worthwhile to teach a student to use her electronic communication aid to complement a teacher, such a behavior could be viewed by classmates negatively, "as browning up." To the contrary (and to adults' discontent), in some classes students without disabilities are valued to the extent that they can insult others without mortally offending them!

The behavior involves the controlled use of an undesired reflex or movement pattern. Once again, this determination requires input from other team members such as OT and PT. In assessing the desirability of any communicative behavior, its relationship to other life functions must be considered. For example, a reflex that results in an arm extending uncontrollably may be useful in indicating a desire for an object. However, once in this position, the same student may now be unable to manipulate the object once it is provided to her, as was the case with Telisha.

Telisha's teacher offered a piece of chalk to her class as she asked for a volunteer to record a response on the blackboard. Telisha responded by turning her head to the right, which in turn triggered a reflex that sent her right arm into extension. The teacher accurately interpreted Telisha's reaching to mean that she wanted the chalk. The teacher called on Telisha and handed her the chalk. However, Telisha was unable to write on the blackboard, while in this reflex pattern, and required full physical assistance from her aide to complete the task.

The behavior is tiring for the student. Students cannot be expected to communicate when the effort associated with doing so exceeds the importance of their reason for communicating. OTs and other team members can provide valuable assessment information related to the choice and placement of switches for activating communication aids and other devices.

The behavior is so specific, or idiosyncratic, to the individual (nonconventional) that it limits the number of people with whom it can be

Student: _____   Date: _____   Time: _____

Activity: _____

BEHAVIORS

- AGGRESSION
- BIZARRE VERBALIZATIONS
- INAPP. ORAL/ANAL BEHAVIOR
- PERSEVERATIVE RITUALS
- SELF-INJURIOUS BEHAVIOR
- SELF STIMULATION
- TANTRUM
- FACIAL EXPRESSION
- GAZE AVERSION
- GAZE / STARING
- GESTURING / POINTING
- HUGGING / KISSING
- MASTURBATION
- OBJECT MANIPULATION
- PROXIMITY POSITIONING
- PUSHING / PULLING
- REACHING / GRABBING
- RUNNING
- TOUCHING
- DELAYED ECHOLALIA
- IMMEDIATE ECHOLALIA
- LAUGHING / GIGGLING
- SCREAM / YELL
- SWEARING
- VERBAL / PHYSICAL THREATS
- WHINING / CRYING
- COMPLEX SIGN / APPROX.
- COMPLEX SPEECH / APPROX.
- ONE WORD SIGN / APPROX.
- ONE WORD SPEECH / APPROX
- PICTURE / WRITTEN WORD

FUNCTIONS

I. INTERACTIVE

A. REQUESTS FOR
- Attention
- Social Interaction
- Play Interactions
- Affection
- Permission to Engage in an Activity
- Action by Receiver
- Assistance
- Information/Clarification
- Objects
- Food

B. NEGATIONS
- Protest
- Refusal
- Cessation

| C. DECLARATIONS/COMMENTS |
| About Events/Actions |
| About Objects/Persons |
| About Errors/Mistakes |
| Affirmation |
| Greeting |
| Humor |
| D. DECLARATIONS ABOUT FEELINGS |
| Anticipation |
| Boredom |
| Confusion |
| Fear |
| Frustration |
| Hurt Feelings |
| Pain |
| Pleasure |
| II. NON-INTERACTIVE |
| A. SELF-REGULATION |
| B. REHEARSAL |
| C. HABITUAL |
| D. RELAXATION/TENSION RELEASE |

FIGURE 4–1

An observational tool for analyzing the communicative functions of behavior. From Donnellan, A., Mirenda, P., Mesaros, R., & Fassbender, L. (1984). Analyzing the communicative functions of aberrant behavior. *Journal of the Association for Persons with Severe Handicaps, 9,* 201–212. With permission.

TABLE 4–2
Circumstances that might indicate the need to modify a student's existing methods of communication

---

1. The behavior is socially unacceptable (e.g., John indicates he would like to join his classmates at a science activity by kicking the child nearest to him).
2. The behavior involves the controlled use of an undesired reflex or movement pattern (e.g., Molly has learned to use her Asymmetric Tonic Neck Reflext [ATNR] to indicate that she wishes to receive materials offered to her by classmates. Through this reflex, her arm and hand extend to the listener).
3. The behavior is tiring for the student (e.g., Sarah is able to point to letters and other symbols directly, yet expends tremendous effort doing so. Her team has decided to use a scanning system instead).
4. The behavior is so specific, or idiosyncratic, to the individual (non-conventional) that it limits the number of children and adults with whom it can be used.
5. The behavior is potentially harmful to the student and/or others (e.g., hitting, biting, pushing, pulling the listener by the arm).
6. The behavior is relatively inefficient (e.g., Tarah was encouraged to point to the materials she desired in art class, rather than making this same request by composing messages on her communication display. Using the earlier method she found that her classmates often grabbed what she might have wanted, before she had the opportunity to indicate her preferences).

Source: Adapted from Reichle, Feeley, & Johnston (1993). Examples have been added.

used. Students need to communicate with classmates, teachers, family members and others in different settings. They will have contact with people who know them well. They will also interact with people who are unfamiliar to them and/or unfamiliar with their methods of communication. Existing (and projected) methods of communication should be assessed relative to their intelligibility to a broad audience of trained as well as untrained listeners. This requires observing students in different settings, with different people. Observations are supplemented with interviews of classmates, teachers, and others to determine the extent to which students' communicative behaviors are understandable.

We have sometimes found it useful to ask teachers and others to independently maintain dictionaries of students' communicative behaviors over a period of several weeks. Entries by different recorders are then compared. We are particularly interested in examining the degree of consensus and disagreement by different recorders as to (1) what constitutes communicative behavior, and (2) what do they perceive to be the intent/meaning of each message. Modes of communication that are associated with a lack of intelligibility are targeted for change. New modes are then introduced so the student can convey the original message/intent more successfully. The instructional setting involves the original recorder and context in which the initial messages were unsuccessful.

The behavior is potentially harmful to the student and/or others. As was illustrated earlier in the case of Shelley, these behaviors may need to be replaced by other methods that are more conventional and socially appropriate.

The behavior is relatively inefficient. This will be determined in context by observing the success of behaviors, listeners' responses, and students' motivation to use the behavior. When students refuse to use communication displays, it may be a clear indication that they have determined the system is not efficient, or no more efficient than methods of communication, such as vocalizations and gestures, they used prior to its introduction (Calculator & Dollaghan, 1982; Calculator & Luchko, 1983).

So far we have looked at present levels of communication relative to (1) how a student communicates, and (2) the purposes and communicative intents of students' messages. We now turn our attention to the final consideration: (3) Whether a student's communicative behavior is intentional.

Intentionality

There are many ways of determining whether students' behaviors are intentional, or simply a reaction to what is happening to and around them. Cirrin and Rowland (1985) suggest observing: (1) direction of the behavior (gaze and body orientation); (2) proximity of the listener; (3) joint focus (alternating gaze between the listener and an object with which the student wishes to engage that listener in some way); (4) substitution of means (the student points to a classmate's snack to indicate that she, too, would like to eat); and (5) persistence of the behavior until the goal is accomplished. Additional factors proposed by Wetherby and Prizant (1990) include: (6) evidence that the student pauses between behaviors (as if waiting for a response from the listener); and (7) altering a behavior when it is not at first successful in producing a desired outcome.

In assessing intentionality, we attempt to determine how aware students are that they can act on and influence others' behavior. As students become more aware of relationships between their actions (e.g., indicating wants and needs, greeting others, requesting clarification, commenting, giving information, and so forth), and others' reactions (acting on those wants and needs, exchanging greetings, clarifying confusing messages, acknowledging, acting on information, and so forth), the effectiveness of their communication increases. This concept is captured nicely in Rowland and Schweigert's (1989) seven levels of communicative competence (Table 4–3).

Examining this table we see that students' communicative abilities may range from preintentional behavior to formal symbolic communication. As we begin along this continuum, the most basic communicative behaviors arise in response to external and internal states such as hunger. These behaviors are often subtle, and may be conveyed in nonconventional ways (crying, changes in posture and tone, aggression, and so forth), leaving ample room for misinterpretation. Students communicating at this level must rely heavily on others to ascribe intentionality to their behavior ("I think he is upset," "I think he wants this," "He hasn't eaten for a long time"; "When was she last repositioned? Perhaps she is uncomfortable"), and then to respond contingently.

Jennfifer's SLP and classroom teacher met to discuss whether or not Jennifer should attend a special assembly. A troupe of visiting artists were performing an environmental play. The teacher had previewed the play and was concerned that the loud, sudden noises; lighting effects; smoke; strange odors; and props would be too much for Jennifer to tolerate.

Rather than excluding her from the assembly, Jennifer was positioned near the front of the audience, beside two friends. Her teacher observed from
continued

TABLE 4–3

Seven levels of communicative competence

Level		Salient Behavior	Examples
I.	Preintentional Behavior	Preintentional or reflexive behavior that expresses *state* of subject. State (e.g., hungry, wet) interpreted by observer.	Cry, coo Facial Expression Postural change
II.	Intentional Behavior (not intentionally communicative)	Behavior is intentional, but is not intentionally communicative. Behavior *functions* to affect observer's behavior since observer infers intent.	Fuss Regard object Reach toward
III.	Nonconventional Presymbolic Communication	Nonconventional gestures are used with *intent* of affecting observer's behavior.	Whine Tug Push away
IV.	Conventional Presymbolic Communication	Conventional gestures are used with intent of affecting observer's behavior.	Alternating gaze Extend object Point/wave Nod/shake head
V.	Concrete Symbolic Communication	Limited use of concrete (iconic) symbols to represent environmental entities. 1:1 correspondence between symbol & referent.	"Natural" gestures Depictive sounds Tangible symbols (objects or pictures)
VI.	Abstract Symbolic Communication	Limited use of abstract (arbitrary) symbols to represent environmental entities. Symbols are used singly.	Spoken words Manual signs Blissymbolics Printed words Brailled words
VII.	Formal Symbolic Communication	Rule-bound use of arbitrary symbol system. Ordered combinations of two or more symbols according to syntactic rules.	Combinations of above abstract symbols

Source: From Rowland, C., & Schweigert, P, (1989). Tangible symbols: Symbolic communication for individuals with multisensory impairments. *Augmentative and Alternative Communication, 5,* 226–234. Reprinted with permission.

> a distance, ready to intervene as necessary. During the performance, classmates responded to Jennifer's changes in expression and body tone by stroking her hair and patting her back. They also issued multiple verbal warnings in anticipation of "wicked scarey parts." Jennifer and her classmates enjoyed the performance greatly.

Proceeding along Rowland and Schweigert's (1989) continuum towards Level VII, Formal Symbolic Communication, we now find students communicating through increasingly intentional, conventional (socially acceptable and generally understood), and abstract methods. Higher levels of communication are associated with access to an increasing number of messages that can be conveyed to more listeners in a greater variety of settings.

Readers should note that no student is excluded as a potential candidate for communication services, using Rowland and Schweigert's (1989) model. It is the content, rather than the availability, of services that change as students exhibit more advanced levels of communicative ability.

■ IDENTIFYING INSTRUCTIONAL GOALS AND OBJECTIVES FOR COMMUNICATION

So far, we have discussed assessment activities related to identifying students' eligibility for communication services, and determining students' present levels of ability. A third primary purpose for conducting communicative assessments for students with severe disabilities is to identify instructional goals and objectives. In Chapter 1, we reviewed best practices for educating students with severe disabilites, presenting partial results of a survey pertaining to the delivery of AAC services in inclusive classrooms. One highly rated best practice suggested that communication goals (should be) individualized for students based on their abilities to meet daily demands.

Discrepancy Analysis

In this procedure, students' communication skills are examined relative to those skills required for full participation in a corresponding activity or event. A variety of observational tools have been suggested for carrying out this activity (Brown et al, 1984; Calculator, 1988; Cipani, 1989; Falvey, 1986; Mirenda & Calculator, 1993). All of these tools require the SLP (and/or others) to begin by compiling an inventory of communication opportunities and demands in different settings. Next, the student's communicative behaviors in these situations are examined. *Discrepancies* that are noted between demands and students' abilities to respond may then be targeted in instruction. Jorgensen (Chapter 2) presents a complete description of this process, along with a case study (Josh) that illustrates its use.

Others suggest conducting a discrepancy analysis by observing nondisabled classmates and recording their communicative behavior in the same settings in which the student's level of participation is to be enhanced (Beukelman & Mirenda, 1992; Calculator & Jorgensen, 1991). Behaviors exhibited by classmates are taught, or an AAC method is introduced, to avail students with severe disabilities the same participation opportunities enjoyed by classmates. These same analyses are used to identify contexts in which communication skills can be fostered and enhanced, as part of a broader curriculum.

Analogue Assessment

Discrepancy analyses provide one source of information for identifying communication goals and objectives. These procedures rely on naturalistic observations of students' communicative behaviors. However, there are times when a particular setting does not provide sufficient opportunities for the SLP and others to observe behaviors of interest. A second procedure, analogue assessment, is particularly useful in these situations (Halle, 1993). Here, the SLP (or others) creates conditions that increase the liklihood that a student will emit a particular behavior. These assessments can be carried out by sabotaging natural routines, as in the following examples.

> When Bill arrives at his table, there are no more seats available (the SLP removed the last chair). The examiner is interested in whether (and how) Bill
> *continued*

solicits his teacher's attention and makes a request (for a chair) to join his group.

Tanya's SLP has programmed (on an electronic communication aid) in the names of several major characters and events from a story that was assigned to the whole class for homework. Immediately before English class, Tanya's aide asks her to hit the keys corresponding to each of these messages, confirming that Tanya is aware of the content and locations of different items on her display.

Once in class, the teacher makes it a point to call on Tanya for answers. The aide documents Tanya's responses to her teacher's questions, indicating whether or not she volunteered or was called on without volunteering. The SLP suggested this activity as a means of assessing Tanya's liklihood of initiating when content necessary to participate in class discussions was programmed on her communication disaplay, and thus available to her.

Maria's teacher wants to know how she responds to other classmates' requests for materials. One day, Maria is given 14 pairs of scissors (needed for math that day). Each child approaches her and verbally requests a scissor. When Maria does not respond, they repeat their request, while also extending their hand towards her. The teacher notes Maria's responses, and then forwards this information to the SLP for later discussion.

During cooking class, Ted's teacher whispers to him that it would be nice if he offered a brownie to a student working alone elsewhere in the room. Ted's (and the student's) response is documented by the teacher. The SLP was paticularly interested in observing whether social overtures from Ted could evoke positive social behaviors from classmates.

Analogue assessments can also be implemented in contrived settings that simulate natural environments. However, caution should be exercised when interpreting these results, given the variability of students' behavior in different settings and resulting problems generalizing results observed in one setting to another.

Dynamic Assessment

A third method of identifying communication goals and objectives relies on dynamic assessment (Olswang & Bain,1991). This procedure enables SLPs and others to determine the extent to which students can benefit from communication instruction. These tasks are useful to carry out in conjunction with discrepancy analyses, as described earlier. Having identified communication problems that are limiting students' participation opportunities and overall inclusion, different variables are manipulated to determine how to best teach corresponding skills to the student.

Returning to the preceding analogue procedure involving Maria, one outcome might be Maria's failing to comply with her classmates' requests for the scissors. The teacher could then seize this moment to provide instruction (e.g., modeling, cueing, prompting Maria). Maria's ability to benefit from this instruction could then be examined by observing her responses to other children's requests for scissors.

Dynamic assessment is also particularly useful when assessing the appropriateness of teachers' and classmates' communicative input to students. For example, students' frequency and accuracy of responding can be examined as others' input is systematically manipulated. Partners can be asked to vary the complexity and redundancy of their speech, to accompany speech with gestures and signs, and to incorporate students' communication systems (e.g., indicating key symbols on a student's communication display as they talk with the general class) in their lectures.

Discrepancy analyses, analogue assessments, and dynamic assessment offer three methods of identifying students' communication and broader educational needs. They are intended as valuable supplements to other forms of observation, interviewing, formal testing and so forth. These and other practices are driven by questions about students' communicative effectiveness, *some* of which are summarized in Table 4–4. Several of these questions are elaborated on below. Questions that are not discussed further have already been addressed elsewhere in this chapter. (Note: Case

TABLE 4–4

Communicative assessment questions that can be used to identify general educational goals and objectives for students with severe disabilities

1. With whom does the student typically interact (classmates, other students, special and general educators, aides, and so forth)?
2. Does the student interact more successfully with some partners than with others?
3. Do partners with whom the student is most and least successful exhibit any consistent characteristics? Can positive qualities be replicated with additional partners (e.g., by using prototypes and other models?) Can negative qualities be extinguished?
4. Is the student spoken to in meaningful, understandable, and culturally and linguistically appropriate ways?
5. What constitutes optimal verbal input for this student (considering language and other abilities).
6. Is the student having a desired impact on others?
7. Is use of the AAC system having a desired impact on others?
8. Does the AAC system reflect the student's preferences (self-determination)?
9. What are the student's attitudes about communication?
10. What types of AAC systems have been tried, and what were the outcomes, with this student? What are the implications?
11. What is the nature and frequency of opportunities for interaction for this student, relative to that experienced by classmates?
12. What messages (form, content, and uses of language) does the student need to be more successful in these settings? (And who is it that these messages should be addressed to?)
13. What supports (e.g., adaptive equipment, personnel, teaching strategies, curriculum modifications) are available and how do they facilitate the student's participation in different settings? (Note: this subject is also addressed in Chapters 2 and 5).
14. Does the student have ready access to AAC and other adaptive equipment?
15. Are there barriers to effective communication (policy and attitudinal)?

studies in the Appendices of this chapter illustrate how these and other assessment questions can be pursued. Footnotes following the Appendices are an additional source of content for assessment procedures.)

With Whom Does the Student Typically Interact? Do Students Interact More Successfully With Some Partners Than With Others? Why?

When a student has a restricted number of people with whom they interact, it may or may not be of their choosing. For example, students who are capable of communicating effectively about a broad range of topics, with familiar as well as unfamiliar people, may be expected to have a large network of potential communication partners. However, this is not necessarily true, particularly if this same student's opportunities for participation are limited.

Assessment activities should always include an inventory of communication partners (classmates, teachers, specialists, family members). Subsequent intervention may then target enhancing a student's effectiveness of communication with these same individuals and/or expanding the pool of potential listeners.

Impact of Communication on Others

In addition to identifying students' communication partners, it is often useful to examine how *effectively* students interact with different partners, in the same and in different settings (Question 2 from Table 4–4). Do partners with whom the student is most and least successful exhibit any consistent characteristics? Can positive qualities (e.g., giving the student sufficient time to respond; providing multiple opportunities to communicate; responding contingently to the student's message) be replicated with additional partners? Can negative qualities (ignoring the student; changing topics initiated by the student; interrupting; rushing the student) be extinguished?

Calculator (1984) advocates identifying people who are particularly successful interacting with the student, referring to these individuals as "prototype" conversational partners. These individuals can be called on to teach (directly, or through modeling) others who are not experiencing comparable levels of success with a particular student.

The National Joint Committee for Meeting the Communicative Needs of Persons With Severe Disabilities (1992) recommended that students with severe disabilities should be spoken to in meaningful, understandable, and culturally and linguistically appropriate ways. A teacher who communicates with a student in an infantilizing manner conveys a lack of respect and low esteem. These qualities may be adopted by classmates. Conversely, teachers who model appropriate methods of interaction contribute to a classroom environment that values all students.

The SLP can determine the optimal nature of verbal input for a particular student. Modifications employed with school-aged children should be limited to those which increase the understandability of a message (e.g., shorter, more redundant utterances, slower rate, referring to immediate, visible objects and events). Affective changes (higher pitched voices, rising intonations, and so forth), may convey a condescending attitude toward the student and should be avoided.

Students' understanding of communication arises and matures through experience. Ideally, students develop an understanding of communication as a means of making things happen. However, when their communicative attempts are ignored or responded to incorrectly, students' motivation to communicate may diminish. Consider the consequences when an adult mistakes a subtle greeting (conveyed by facial grimacing) as an indication that the student wants to be left alone. The adult walks away from the student who has attempted to engage him in interaction. Vicker (1985) discusses procedures for teaching others to recognize and respond to students' messages, thus expanding the number of conversational partners.

Impact Relative to Choice of Communicative Mode

The impact of students' communicative attempts on others may also vary depending on students' methods of communication. AAC systems are often suggested as means of enhancing commmunicative effectiveness. However, what happens when AAC systems do not enhance communication significantly?

Calculator and Dollaghan (1982) described students who were no more successful when they relied on their communication boards, than when they used "ambiguous" methods of communication. Similarly these students were as likely to resolve communication breakdowns by resorting to unintelligible vocalizations and ambiguous gestures, as they were to employ their communication boards in these situations. Again, no advantages were associated with using the communication boards, relative to impact on classmates and teachers. It was thus not surprising to the investigators that these teachers did not encourage the students to use their communication boards in their everyday interactions.

Self-determination

Subjects in the Calculator and Dollaghan (1982) investigation exercised their right to choose their methods of communication. While a student may be an excellent candidate for a particular AAC device, this aid will be of no value if the student is unwilling to use it. In assessing students' communication needs, it is imperative to delineate their (and others') preferences for one mode of communication relative to others. Preferences must be respected, once individuals have been informed of the full range of uses associated with each system.

This is particularly important for students at the secondary level. These students may benefit from training that focuses on enhancing their skills as consumers, encouraging them to make their own decisions about what services they do and do not need. (Note: The topic of self-determination is discussed in Chapter 6.)

Similarly, students' attitudes towards communication (in general as well as with particular partners) must be assessed. By the time students reach first grade (much less secondary school) they have often received extensive communication training. In that time, they (and their families) have been subjected to practices that may be motivated more by particular educators' preferences and whims, and "new" trends and advances, than their actual needs.

Over the past 17 years, I have encountered numerous students whose intervention histories included stints with signs/gestures (moving from one system to another), communication boards, electronic aids, speech, more sign, more aids, speech, more communication boards, more signs. By the time I entered the picture, they (and their families) were understandably leery of the prospects of still another addendum to a history of fragmented instruction.

Prior to moving ahead, it is imperative that we describe the content and relative effectiveness of past attempts to address students' communication needs. This information can be obtained through interview (students, parents, teachers [past and present]) and comprehensive review of students' files. Unfortunately, schools often divide students' folders, retaining recent information in one location while housing outdated information elsewhere. This latter information is critical in helping us to understand students' current communication abilities and preferences.

What Opportunities for Interaction Exist Presently?

This assessment may begin with an examination of students' opportunities to make choices and to indicate preferences in different settings. Classmates without disabilities typically have multiple opportunities to make choices and indicate preferences. Some of these choices are presented overtly by their teachers. For example, students may be instructed to select a book from a reading center during silent reading or determine a role for each member of their group prior to undertaking a cooperative learning task. More often, such opportunities are covert, for example, students select where (and how) they wish to sit, how long (within reasonable limits) they will "hang out" in the cafeteria before going outside, which writing utensils (pencils and pens) they will use, to whom they will direct requests for assistance, and so forth.

Unlike their classmates, students with severe disablities often find choices being delegated (overtly) by others. While their classmates select media they wish to use to draw a picture, a student with severe disabilities may be expected to choose from two or more pre-selected choices presented by another.

Opportunities to indicate preferences and choices can be assessed using discrepancy analyses and other procedures already discussed in this chapter. These same procedures can be used to identify ways of modifying activities to foster more of these opportunities.

Access to AAC and Other Adaptive Equipment

Students' opportunities to interact depend, in part, on the accessibility of AAC and other adaptive equipment. Equipment should be present and in good working condition. When equipment is not being used, it is critical that we determine the reason (inadequate training, lack of success, and so forth).

Opportunities for communication may also be limited by different types of barriers that need to be identified (Beukelman & Mirenda, 1992; Jones, Beukelman, & Hiatt, 1992). For example, policies such as requiring all AAC systems to remain at school, where they are not to be used by anyone but the designated student, may need to be reexamined. The assessment should also identify what Jones et al. (1992) refer to as attitudinal barriers posed by educators and others toward students, technology, inclusion, and so forth.

■□ SUMMARY

This chapter has presented a variety of assessment principles and procedures for students with severe disabilities to determine their eligibility for communication services, present levels of ability, and instructional needs. All of these procedures examine communication relative to broader concerns related to interaction, participation, and inclusion. This material serves as an introduction to Chapter 5, where additional intervention procedures are described.

■□ FROM THEORY TO PRACTICE

The Appendices which follow provide examples of how many of the principles discussed above can be incorporated into an assessment plan and, more specifically, a resulting report. Six reports are presented, all drawn from the clinical files of the author.

Cases presented were selected from over 100 files. Students represent a variety of grade levels (preschool [e.g., Ally], early elementary [Crystal and Ivan], middle school [Ariel and Ann], and high school [Sam]); placements (integrated part-time to fully included); communication abilities (prelinguistic to symbolic); and communication systems.

Two students (Ally and Sam) relied primarily on preverbal gestures and vocalizations; one used facilitated communication (Ariel); one (Ann) used a combination of picture boards, gestures, and other communication modes; one spoke (Crystal); and one (Ivan) used a combination of unaided (vocalizations, gestures, and signs) and aided (communication boards and electronic communication devices) modes.

Each report is unedited with the exception that identifying information has been deleted. Footnotes (as superscripts) have been added to indicate that a particular assessment principle (listed at the end of the chapter) is being demonstrated. Readers are encouraged to identify such principles on their own, particularly as they peruse Ann's report (where footnotes have purposely been deleted).

■□ REFERENCES

American Speech-Language-Hearing Association Committee on Language Learning Disorders. (1989). Report on issues in determining eligibility for language intervention. *Asha, 31*(3), 113–118.

Beukelman, D., & Mirenda, P. (1992). *Augmentative and Alternative Communication: Management of Severe Communication Disorders in Children and Adults.* Baltimore: Paul H. Brookes Publishing Company.

Brown, L., Shiraga, B., York, J., Zanella,K., & Rogan, K. (1984). *The discrepancy analysis technique in programs for students with severe handicaps.* Madison, WI: University of Wisconsin-Madison and Madison Metropolitan School District.

Calculator, S. (1984). Prelinguistic development. In W. Perkins (Ed.), *Language handicaps in children* (pp. 63–71). New York: Thieme-Stratton.

Calculator, S. (1988). Promoting the acquisition and generalization of conversational skills by individuals with severe handicaps. *Augmentative and Alternative Communication, 4,* 94–103.

Calculator, S., & Dollaghan, C. (1982). The use of communication boards in a residential setting. *Journal of Speech and Hearing Disorders, 14,* 281–287.

Calculator, S., & Jorgensen, C. (1991). Integrating AAC instruction into regular education settings: Expounding on best practices. *Augmentative and Alternative Communication, 7,* 204–214.

Calculator, S., & Luchko, C. (1983). Evaluating the effectiveness of a communication board training program. *Journal of Speech and Hearing Disorders, 48,* 185–192.

Casby, M. (1992). The cognitive hypothesis and its influence on speech-language services in schools. *Language, Speech, and Hearing Services in Schools, 23,* 198–202.

Cipani, E. (1989). Providing language consultation in the natural context: A model for delivery of services. *Mental Retardation, 27,* 317–324.

Cirrin, F., & Rowland, C. (1985). Communication assessment of nonverbal youths with severe/profound mental retardation. *Mental Retardation, 23,* 52–62.

Cole, K., Dale, P., & Mills, P. (1990). Defining language delay in young children by cognitive referencing: Are we saying more than we know? *Applied Psycholinguistics, 11,* 291–302.

Donnellan, A., Mirenda, P., Mesaros, R., & Fassbender, L. (1984). Analyzing the communicative functions of aberrant behavior. *Journal of the Association for Persons with Severe Handicaps, 9,* 201–212.

Falvey, M. (1986). *Community Based Curriculum: Instructional Strategies for Students with Severe Handicaps.* Baltimore: Paul H. Brookes.

Halle, J. (1993). Innovative assessment measures and practices designed with the goal of achieving functional communication and integration. In L. Kupper (Ed.), *The Second National Symposium on Effective Communication for Children and Youth with Severe Disabilities: A Vision for the Future* (pp. 201–251). McLean, VA: Interstate Research Associates, Inc.

Jones, R., Beukelman, D., & Hiatt, E. (1992). Educational integration of students who use augmentative and alternative communication systems. *Seminars in Speech and Language, 13*(2), 120–129.

Leary, J., & Boscardin, M. (1992). Ethics and efficacy of verbal testing of nonverbal children: A case study. *Remedial and Special Education, 13* (4), 52–61.

Miller, J., Chapman, R., & Bedrosian, J. (1977). Defining developmentally disabled subjects for research: The relationship between etiology, cognitive development, and language and communicative performance. Paper presented at the Second Annual Boston University Conference on Language Development, Boston, MA.

Mirenda, P., & Calculator, S. (1993). Enhancing curricula design. *Clinics in Communication Disorders, 3,* 43–58.

National Joint Committee for Meeting the Communicative Needs of Persons with Severe Disabilities. (1992). Guidelines for meeting the communication needs of persons with severe disabilities. *Asha, 34*(3), (Suppl. 7), 1–8.

Noonan, M.J., & Siegel-Causey, E. (1990). Special needs of students with severe handicaps. In L. McCormick & R. Schiefelbusch (Eds.). *Early language intervention: An introduction* (2nd ed., pp. 383–425). Columbus, OH: Merrill Publishing Company.

Olswang, L., & Bain, B. (1991). When to recommend intervention. *Language,Speech, and Hearing Services in Schools, 22,* 255–263.

Reichle, J., Feeley, K., & Johnston, S. (1993). Communication intervention for persons with severe and profound disabilities. *Clinics in Communication Disorders, 3,* 7–30.

Richard, N., & Schiefelbusch, R. (1990). Assessment. In L. McCormick & R. Schiefelbusch (Eds.). 109–141. *Early language intervention: An Introduction,* (2nd ed., pp. 109–141). Columbus, OH: Merrill Publishing Company.

Rowland, C., & Schweigert, P. (1989). Tangible symbols: Symbolic communication for individuals with multisensory impairments. *Augmentative and Alternative Communication, 5,* 226–234.

Vicker, B. (1985). *Recognizing and enhancing the communication skills of your group home clients.* Bloomington: Indiana University Developmental Training Center.

Wetherby, A., & Prizant, B. (1990). *Communicative and symbolic behavior scales—Research edition.* Chicago: Riverside Publishing.

■□ APPENDIX A

■□ ALLY

Speech-Language Consultation

Background Information

Ally's educational, medical, and related background information have been well documented elsewhere (see educational folder).

Thus, the present report will concentrate on suggestions previewed with team members at the conclusion of my April 16th visit.[1]

Presently, Ally appears to receive the majority of her services from Physical Therapy, Occupational Therapy (Ginny), and Speech-Language (Elly). She is supported 1:1 by Toni, who accurately refers to herself as a nurse, teacher, special educator, friend (of Ally's), . . . Toni has primary responsibility for assisting Ally in therapy, carryover of program objectives, and supporting her in the preschool program.[2]

Ally attends the preschool approximately 45 minutes each day, during which there do not appear to be any formal academic expectations of her. The team described this as a situation in which the primary objectives relate to providing Ally with opportunities to be around peers, benefit from socialization, and become more tolerant of stimulation (human and other) to and around her.[3]

The team indicated that Ally is the first child with severe disabilities (of her magnitude) to be integrated at the school. The primary reason for this consultation was to observe the program and then discuss suggestions for restructuring her program in the future. Suggestions which follow thus relate both to program content and service delivery.

Suggestions/Recommendations

Ally is a young girl with tremendous needs. Her team has expended great effort in developing a program at Still Water since her arrival this past January. The current focus on related services might now be broadened to embrace more of an environmentally referenced (as opposed to a discipline-referenced) educational plan. This concept was reviewed with several team members at the conclusion of my visit. For example, rather than looking at speech/language and developmental milestones which might be addressed at this time, the team might instead consider addressing communicative behaviors which would enhance Ally's participation in the preschool program.[4] Similarly, efforts to maintain and enhance range of motion might correspond to functional, in-class routines in which these same abilities are necessary and can be reinforced naturally.[4] Along these same lines, adaptive equipment such as the supine stander should be introduced in class as a means of supporting participation in a given activity [preferably one in which participation requires other students to assume an upright position as well].[4]

Ally would benefit greatly from communication training which is systematically integrated within a broader educational program. The underlying theme would be to continually expand her currently restricted range of communicative and other responses, tieing such behaviors to the corresponding contexts in which they are useful, via the matrix.[5]

In moving to such a program, the following might be considered by the team:

1. Terry continues to be a tremendous source of nurturance and instructional support for Ally. In observing Ally in class, and subsequently meeting with the preschool teacher, I was also struck by the high level of acceptance communicated by this teacher and other students towards Ally. A primary component which is lacking at this point is evidence of systematic programming and educational expectations made of Ally within the classroom.[4]

During my visit, I introduced the notion of Matrixing as a means of generating functional goals, and then addressing these same goals in various natural settings (Elly has a copy of these and all other materials noted in the present report). Through matrixing, a person (Toni, the teacher, a classmate, the speech-language pathologist) is designated to address a particular objective (e.g., turning and establishing eye contact with a listener, purposeful reaching, shifting gaze from one speaker to another, requesting continuance of an activity which has been temporarily terminated) in conjunction with a regularly scheduled classroom activity (e.g., free play, calendar, activity centers, gym, snack . . .).[4]

2. In order to implement such a program, it would be beneficial to identify a program manager/consultant/integration specialist whose primary responsibility might consist of teaming with the classroom teacher and others in order to assist in developing daily schedules, confer with the teacher and Toni, develop means of documenting objectives and progress, review progress regularly, and revise programs as necessary. Further information about the roles such a person might fulfill can be obtained by contacting the New Hampshire Statewide Systems Change Project and requesting to speak with either Carol or Cheryl, both of whom have had extensive experience with this model of service delivery.[2]

3. In addition to matrixing, additional ideas for goals (along with methods of integrating such goals into ongoing educational programs) can be found in the C.O.A.C.H. (Giangreco et al.), which is published by Brookes, Inc. This device is intended as a means of developing a child's program, with primary emphasis placed on parental input. The procedure requires approximately 2 hours to administer. When implemented in conjunction with tools such as the Functional Analysis of Opportunities to Participate in Regular School Activities (Calculator & Jorgensen, 1991), and the Classroom Activity Analysis Worksheet (Note: Elly has copies), the team will have an adequate basis for prioritizing goals.[4]

Finally, the vision consultant[2] might be contacted for information pertaining to the Van Dijk program. These procedures have been found to be useful in developing a rudimentary set of communicative and intentional behaviors, beginning with responses that are already in the child's repertoire. Strategies (e.g., object calendars and anticipation shelves) related to the promotion of anticipatory responses might also be useful in easing transitions from activity to activity and forming a rudimentary communication system for Ally.

4. Positioning will continue to be a major factor in promoting normal neuromuscular functioning, as well as enhancing participation opportunities. The Physical Therapist can be a major source of information to other team members in identifying and using adaptive equipment, following observation of Ally in classroom and related environments.[4]

5. Toni indicated that Ally often has difficulties with transitions from activity to activity. The Occupational Therapist may be a good resource in this regard, recommending techniques through which such transitions can be eased (e.g., desensitization, stimulus presentation, and so forth).

6. Teachers and others need to be aware of the amount and complexity of language addressed to Ally, as well as speaking rate.[6] The speech-language pathologist might provide inservice instruction to other team members regarding methods of simplifying their language and thus enhancing responsiveness on the part of Ally.

7. The district might consider sponsoring a workshop on inclusive schooling/techniques for integrating children with severe disabilities into regular education. Again, depending on the needs and objectives, I would be happy to assist with such a program and/or suggest the names of alternative speakers.[4]

8. Please feel free to contact me if I can be of any further assistance. Ally is indeed fortunate to have surrounded herself with such a caring circle of friends and professionals. I applaud your efforts.

Stephen N. Calculator, Ph.D., CCC-Sp.
Consulting Speech-Language Pathologist

■□ APPENDIX B

■□ ARIEL

Speech-Language Consultation

Background

As Ariel's history is well documented elsewhere, the reader is referred to her educational file for information pertaining to prior
evaluations and school placements. The present assessment was
conducted in order to assist Ariel's team in identifying appropriate communication objectives, and means of delivering these services most effectively. More specifically, the team sought input
regarding (1) the feasibility of Facilitated Communication, and (2)
other methods of augmentative communication for Ariel.

Mary (Institute on Developmental Disabilities—Statewide Systems Change Project) had reported that Ariel was an adept communicator who was able to use an alphabet board to engage in
conversations with her. She has visited Ariel at home one to two
times each week for the past few months, initially encouraging her
use of facilitated communication with a letter board, then on a
Macintosh computer, and most recently with a Canon Communicator. The latter device is a dedicated communication aid which
permits its user to spell messages which, in turn, are printed out
on a ticker tape which emerges from one side of the device. Mary
has compiled a journal of messages produced by Ariel with the
Canon and other devices.

According to Mary, Ariel maintains and shifts topics of conversation using syntactically complete phrases. Ariel is able to
converse about a wide range of past, present, and future events;
shares ideas and feelings; and can hold her own as a conversational partner. Additional reporting by Ariel's mother, Marge, con-
firmed Ariel's ability to encode messages on the letter board.
However, Marge indicated that Ariel's messages to her were simplified (one and two word utterances), relative to the types of interactions she observed her daughter engaging in with Mary.

Ariel has been a 9th grade student at Wadell Junior High
School since January, 1991. She currently attends a program designed for students with developmental disabilities, with multiple
opportunities for integration with typical students throughout the

day. Her primary teacher, Linda Gage, oversees both aspects (the resource room and the regular classroom) of Ariel's educational program, consulting to teachers and Aides who, in turn, provide much of the actual instruction.[2]

Prior to arriving at Wadell, Ariel participated in the SAM Program at Pinta Middle School. Many of her present communication objectives (e.g., the use of an object calendar to cue her as to her daily schedule, the use of natural gestures, choice making, indications of preference, etc.) are based on an assessment conducted by this examiner on 4/19/90 at this previous placement. The appropriateness of these recommendations has now been called into question in light of Ariel's propensity for facilitated communication.

Ariel was recently observed by Cheryl Jorgensen 5/9/91, who offered the following suggestions to staff:

1. Increase opportunities for integration, with a more natural flow from class to class rather than moving to and from her self-contained program.
2. Identify an alternate home room.[2]
3. Increased opportunities to interact with typical children, in and out of class.[2]
4. Shift the Aides' roles from primary interactional partner (for Ariel) to facilitator of interactions between Ariel and her teachers, classmates, and others.[7]
5. In-service training of Ariel's teachers as to her abilities and needs, and promoting their more active participation as team members.

In addition to the above recommendations, Dr. Jorgensen alluded to several other modifications in Ariel's present program, within the text of her report. I have attempted to pull these out, and list them below:

6. Staff should refrain from providing an over abundance of physical prompts and cues. Specifically, Dr. Jorgensen encouraged staff to give Ariel the opportunity to do things herself, offering help only to the extent to which it is needed.[6]
7. When interacting with Ariel, it was felt useful to approach her at eye level and then speak with her in a relatively quiet and even tone of voice. These behaviors were found to facilitate attending and listening skills.[6]

8. Inform Ariel's teachers about the meaning of her vocal-izations.[6]
9. Incorporate the results of the COACH (administered by Jorgensen to Marge) into Ariel's educational program. Through the COACH, Marge was helped to identify and then prioritize her goals for Ariel.
10. Identify opportunities for participation (through modifi-cations in curricula, support personnel, instructional strategies) in different classes. This necessitates increased collaboration between regular and special educators.[8]
11. Initiate "Circles of Friends" activities to broaden peer supports available to Ariel.[2]
12. Finally, as part of this assessment I had the opportunity to visit Ariel at home and chat with she, her mother, and Mary. During this visit (and a follow-up phone call), Marge expressed interest in finding an electronic com-munication aid (other than the Canon Communicator) which would give Ariel access to speech synthesis.

Summary

In attempting to design a quality educational program for a child with challenging needs, many factors can enhance this process considerably. Some which come to mind include:

1. Involved parents who take an interest and direct role in their child's educational program, initiate contact with the school, clearly communicate their ideas and feelings to the rest of the team.[4]
2. Team members who are committed to providing an appro-priate (and best) educational program for the child. Un-fortunately, the desire for quality is often accompanied by feelings of inadequacy, failing, etc. as individuals always get the feeling that they could and should be doing more things, better, more consistently.[4]
3. Advocates for the student and his/her family who can support the parent in expressing priorities, dreams, etc.[4]
4. Outside consultants who can offer additional expertise to the team, from an objective point of view.[4]
5. A student whose appearance and nature inspire all around him/her to do their very best.[4]

6. General direction from a broader source (e.g., State Dept. of Education) as to the match between the child's program and effective educational services in more of a generic sense.[4]

In the case of Ariel and her Team, all of these factors clearly exist. It is apparent that all who come in contact with Ariel and her extended family operate in Ariel's best interests. Problems arise, however when those best interests represent conflicting ideas, opinions, philosophies, and experiences. The inevitable result is a breakdown in communication among team members, hostilities, doubts, fears, exasperation.[4]

At this time, I feel it is most essential to **stop** what we are doing, think, and then agree upon **one** course of action for Ariel.[4] The remainder of this report will be devoted to suggestions of my own (hopefully, no one will perceive these as additional baggage to be heaped on what has already become an unmanageable number of ideas from others). The suggestions reflect what I believe to be consensus among all team members,[1] and assent of Ariel, that communication training should:

1. Promote interactions between Ariel and her teachers.[8]
2. Promote interactions between Ariel and her classmates.[8]
3. Provide means by which Ariel is able to more actively participate in classroom activities.[5]
4. Provide means by which Ariel can share feelings and emotions with others.[5]
5. Provide means by which Ariel can have a greater say with respect to her likes and dislikes, choices, preferences, etc.[5]
6. Nurture the development of relationships between Ariel and others. In part, this requires a means by which Ariel can inform others of **who** she is, what is she all about, what is special about her as a person.[7]

The suggestions that follow should be discussed among team members, and Ariel (as her mother deems appropriate).

1. Facilitated Communication

During my visit to Ariel's home, I observed her using the Canon Communicator with Mary. I can now conclude, with minimal reservations, that Ariel does indeed use the Canon to spell messages in a conversational format. The efficacy of facilitated communication remains controversial. However, the abundance of misspellings, topic changes, and offering of content unknown to

Mary can not lead to any conclusion other than the fact that Ariel is (with Facilitated Communication) able to express herself. The difficulty lies in Ariel's exhibiting these same skills with others. The lack of generalization should not be blamed on others' inadequacies any moreso than a weakness on the part of Ariel.

All individuals vary their methods of communication depending on the person with whom they are interacting. A plausible explanation for Ariel's behavior may be that a **necessary precursor** to the effective use of Facilitated Communiation is the presence of a valued and special (at this time undefined) relationship between the facilitator and the facilitatee
(I'm taking license with terminology here).

Marge has clearly stated that she does not feel it is in Ariel's best interests to introduce Facilitated Communication at school at this time. I share her concerns that such action would be doomed for failure and misinterpretation. Central to this technique is adapting a posture in which the student feels valued and supported, convinced that their partner views them as an intelligent individual with much to offer (Recall the earlier discussion about precursors to this technique). Staff at school can lay the groundwork for the introduction of Facilitated Communication in several ways.

1. Identify persons who will be future facilitators through the "Circles of Friends," teacher training, and other initiatives suggested by Cheryl Jorgensen.[7]

2. Promote interactions between Ariel and classmates, teachers, etc. The use of cooperative learning and similar collaborative learning ventures will enhance Ariel's feelings about others, and vice-versa.[8] A primary role of the Aide is to facilitate these interactions, releasing her role to others (training, monitoring, and stepping in as needed).[7]

3. Prepare a 15 minute videotape (with Ariel's permission) of Facilitated Communication with Ariel and (1) Her mother; (2) Mary; (3) A relatively unfamiliar partner. This tape could demonstrate ability and variability of Ariel's interactions relative to different partners. Some tips on **how** to Facilitate might be included at the end of the tape as well.[6] The tape might be shown now, and in the future, to Ariel's teachers and those participating in her Circle of Friends.[9] One purpose would be to effect changes in others' expectations of and attitudes about Ariel; reconsideration of academic goals; assessments of how much Ariel derives academically from inclusion; etc.

Facilitated Communication provides an immediate outlet through which Ariel can relate feelings, opinions etc. It would be ideal if this outlet was available with persons beyond Mary and Marge, to include friends and others. Mary has indicated her willingness to teach others - I would strongly recommend accepting this offer in conjunction with other efforts to develop relationships between Ariel and others. Initially, perhaps a single friend or two could be targeted for training.[9]

Cindy (speech-language pathologist) is very willing and interested in promoting the use of Facilitated Communication once given the go ahead. The team might consider Cindy's introducing facilitated communication to a peer of Ariel's, in the form of yes/no responses.[7] The same letter board used at home could be employed, yet all questions would take the form of yes/no responses. The questions themselves would be agreed upon by the peer and Cindy, in advance, to avoid asking tutorial questions. Ariel has demonstrated an unwillingness to "perform." If Facilitated Communication is introduced, it must be done so in a relevant and meaningful fashion, rather than as a program goal which is addressed non-meaningfully through activities such as asking questions to which the listener already knows the answer.

The Guidance Counselor would be a logical person to develop expertise in Facilitated Communication (and a relationship with Ariel). A designated time might be set aside in which Ariel can communicate confidentially with the counselor. The counselor might relate to the team her impressions regarding Ariel's (and her joint) abilities to share information during sessions, while not divulging the actual content of these sessions.[2]

2.   Augmentative Communication

Like facilitated communication, the efficacy of augmentative communication rests with the child's appreciating the types of access such systems afford. Given the relationships are not valued, or the interactions afforded are not substantially different than those occurring without the device, it is unlikely that the device will be valued (or used).[5] Instead, it is discarded as one of a parade of techniques which are sequentially introduced. (for Ariel, we have seen sign language, natural gestures, Amer-Ind, object boards, a Wolf, Touch Talker . . .). For these reasons I would not search out another device at this time. Instead, concentrate on the underpinnings of all communication: participation, opportunities, access.[10]

Communication will be of value only to the extent to which it promotes Ariel's active, more independent, and voluntary participation in and out of school. At the same time, the driving force behind communication and other aspects of Ariel's educational program should be consistent with concurrent efforts related to developing her Circle of Friends.[4]

Ariel is an affectionate, attractive, intelligent young woman who has much to teach all of us. In the process, I am afraid that we will always fight back feelings that we are not doing the right things, not doing enough, etc. It is essential that her team pull together and present a unified, unquestionable source of positive support for Ariel. The potential of moving ahead for Ariel and the rest of us is too attractive to pass by.

1. In reviewing her file, I was unable to find information pertaining to the extent of her vision. Reference is made to her being legally blind, secondary to bilateral optic nerve hyperplasia. It is also suggested that Ariel may hold her head in unusual positions in order to focus (she may see best from the top of one eye and the bottom of the other). It is essential that the team (and all persons working with Ariel) have a clear understanding of just how much functional vision Ariel possesses and how such vision can be maximized (compensatory behaviors; instructional modifications; changes in teaching style). Since Glorie, the vision consultant, is already involved in Ariel's program, she would be a logical person to speak with staff about the nature of Ariel's vision problems and their social-educational implications.[2] An ongoing consultative role may certainly be called for as well. Gloria may also be in a position to recommend further testing. It is obvious that Ariel has learned to compensate effectively for vision problems she possesses (as demonstrated by her ability to access letter boards, the Canon Communicator; get around in her environment). Less obvious are methods of assisting her through alternate teaching strategies, resources, etc.

2. Speech-language services remain highly warranted at this time. Services should be provided consultatively. Cindy might best consult with Linda [the teacher] who, in turn, assumes responsibility for assuring that Aides are integrating communication objectives while promoting social interactions between Ariel and classmates.[7]

The Activitiy Matrix, and related procedures, will provide a means of systematically determining which objectives will be addressed when, necessary antecedents, behaviors and consequences, etc. Progress and other program decisions can be discussed during Cindy's consultations to the program.[3] Cindy might also spend some time modeling desired techniques for Aides and other direct service providers. Initially, we are probably looking at relatively intense involvement for Cindy as she identifies who will be carrying out the various communication objectives, and provides the necessary training, modeling, and feedback to get these programs going (we may be talking about two hours per day, for a total of five days). Once the programs are up and going, however, the primary responsibility for monitoring and modifying would fall in Linda's hands, with consultation from Cindy (who may then drop back to 2 units per week).[6,7]

3. Cindy might also provide training to peers and the Guidance Counselor relative to the use of Facilitated Communication (as described above). Once again, the timing here must respect Marge's feelings regarding this matter, along with the necessary groundwork which must precede such training (developing friends, enhancing attitudes of others, etc.).

4. The use of backward chaining (Do all but the last step, then have Ariel complete the task [e.g., threading the sewing machine]) and partial participation (with greatly reduced reliance on full physical prompting) would increase Ariel's levels of participation in regular classes. Regular educators and Aides could be instructed in the use of such strategies by Linda. Cheryl Jorgensen's report provides multiple examples of partial participation and methods of identifying relevant instructional goals in regular classes.[11]

5. Decrease reliance on the Aides while increasing collaboration with classmates (e.g., in getting from class to class, activity to activity within classes; step to step within activities). The Aides can be a very valuable support to the class (of which Ariel is a member).[2]

6. Linda might inform teachers and others as to the meaning of Ariel's various behaviors, and the potential for misinterpretation. For example, when Ariel giggles it does not necessarily mean that she is happy. Instead, this is often a sign that she is anxious and frustrated and requires clarification of what is being expected of her and why. Once again, the Guidance Counselor may play a role here as well. Similarly, while Ariel often appears to be looking away from a particular activity, in reality she may be compensating for visual and other disabilities. A lack of attending behavior should not be misinterpreted as a lack of attending or interest.[2,6]

7. Teachers have noted that Ariel performs better, and appears more content, in small group activities than in large group (more individualized) classes. Once again, this has strong implications regarding the types of classes in which to involve Ariel and/or the way in which her classes are structured (e.g., teaching styles; use of cooperative learning and other techniques which promote peer involvement).[11]

8. Systematically identify, target, and reinforce communication behaviors which are relevant to Ariel's participation in various classes, in those classes. Again, Cheryl provides several examples of how such behaviors can be identified using a process known as discrepancy analysis. Such content should be incorporated into the Activity Matrices, with necessary consultation provided by Linda and, to a lesser extent, Cindy. The team might consider requesting Cheryl or myself return in order to teach others (e.g., Linda and the director of special education) how to use such tools to identify short-term objectives for Ariel.

Please feel free to contact me if I can be of any further assistance. I hope that this report clarifies and provides bridges among the separate ideas, orientations, and strategies which comprise Ariel's program.

Sincerely,

Stephen N. Calculator, Ph.D.
Consulting Speech-Language Pathologist

■□ APPENDIX C

■□ CRYSTAL

Speech-Language Consultation

Background Information

Crystal was referred for speech-language consultation by Joan (special education teacher). The primary purpose of this consultation was to offer suggestions to Crystal's 1st grade team relative to future communication training. The team was particularly interested

in determining Crystal's candidacy for augmentative communication instruction, in light of her highly unintelligible speech. Background information is covered adequately elsewhere in her file and
will thus not be reiterated here.

Present Findings

The present assessment consisted of a combination of formal
and informal procedures designed to identify current communication skills and implications for subsequent instruction. The majority of testing was conducted in Crystal's home in the presence of
her mother, brother, and a neighborhood friend.[12] Additional information was gathered by observing Crystal in her classroom,
discussions with her Kindergarten teacher (Jana), speech-language
therapist (Nicki), instructional aide (Mary), mother, and Joan.

The assessment began with informal participant observation
of Crystal during play with her brother and a friend. Crystal initiated and responded to others' messages, sustained topics of conversation, offered new information, related recent experiences,
clarified messages upon her listeners' requests. The latter usually
consisted of repetitions of her previously unsuccessful messages.
When these revisions were again unsuccessful, she often refused
to try again.

At times, Crystal appeared embarassed by her inability to be
understood, withdrawing from and breaking eye contact with her
listener. Speech was more plentiful, intelligible, and louder in
unstructured situations in which it was not a focal point. As we
shifted to formal contexts (e.g., seat work and testing), intelligibility diminished significantly, loudness decreased to the point that
she was barely audible at times, amount of talking, particularly initiations, dropped significantly, and she adopted a shy and hesitant
demeanor.[11] This was in contrast to her mother's reports that she is
such a chatterbox, and her speech occasionally so loud, that she is
sometimes asked to quiet down in the car during family excursions.

Spontaneous messages were generally limited to 3–5 words in
length. Her speech (spontaneous, as well as that evoked through
formal testing) was characterized as follows: *Articulation*: Most significant problems are noted on attempts at rapid alternating movement (i.e., dysdiadichokinesia seen in attempts to utter /pataka/,
/lalalala/, /tatatata/, /takatakataka/, /pattycake/ . . .). With increasing rate, precision decreased, groping increased, and Crystal grew
more anxious. Articulation was imprecise, secondary to distorted

vowels (often resulting from inordinate prolongation), inadequate force of contact, diminished speed, problems with timing, mono-pitch (excess and equal stress), monoloudness (some excess and equal loudness), and scanning speech (each word in a sentence is uttered on a complete pitch contour with equal stress).

Results of a Khan-Lewis Phonological Analysis revealed mul-tiple processes effecting Crystal's speech. This test involves whole word analysis of the Goldman-Fristoe Test of Articulation, with errors then examined for systematicity. Crystal exhibited "excessive" use of final consonant deletion (an early process), velar fronting and stridency deletion (intermediate processes), and cluster sim-plification (a relatively late process). [Note: A copy of the test pro-tocol is enclosed to provide examples of these various errors]. **Note to readers: key staff at Crystal's school were familiarized with this terminology prior to receiving this report!** Moderate use of syllable reduction and palatal fronting (early processes) as well as stopping of fricatives (a late inhibited process) were also noted.

Intelligibility was examined formally using the Assessment of Intelligibility of Dysarthric Speech. One of a field of 12 possible choices (printed words) was pointed to and Crystal's mother whis-pered the stimulus word in Crystal's ear. Crystal then repeated the stimulus word on audiotape. The first 34 items were administered, then testing was terminated as Crystal grew increasingly anxious and began to withdraw. It was felt that the partial test provided a sufficient sample of speech. Mary, Crystal's aide at school, was asked to transcribe each of the 34 words from audiotape. None of the words were correctly transcribed (0% intelligible for isolated words out of context). Mary then attempted to select which word (of 12 choices) Crystal was attempting over the same succession of 34 responses. This task resulted in a score of 24% intelligible.

Subsequent discussion with Mary revealed that she relies heavily on context and watching Crystal's face to understand her better. Without contextual cues (e.g., knowledge of what was go-ing on at the time of the utterance, knowledge of topic, etc.), she estimated Crystal's speech to be approximately 50% intelligible. A less familiar listener, Nicki , estimated her speech to be less than 25% intelligible when the context was unknown. Conversely, Crystal's mother indicated that she understands most (around 90%) of Crystal's conversational speech, estimating her husband has a bit more difficulty with Crystal (approximately 75% intelligible).[13]

In examining these results, findings are consistent with ataxic dysarthria (secondary to cerebellar lesion). Speech problems are due largely to overall hypotonia, dysmetria (problems guaging the force, speed and direction of movement, undershooting of movements), and decomposition of movement (scanning speech).

Respiration: Crystal appears to exhibit limited breath support for speech. Breathing is shallow and vital capacity (amount of air that can be exhaled following inhalation) is diminished, resulting in abbreviated length of utterances and inadequate loudness. Crystal can take in greater volumes of air, when asked to, yet often begins with low volumes of air. Breath support is further limited by air escape (e.g., nares flare during blowing, suggesting velarpharyngeal closure difficulty with escapage of air out of the nose).

Voice: Pitch appears low and is accompanied by monoloudness and monopitch, as cited earlier. Voicing errors (replacing sounds with their voiced/voiceless cognates) are more common in connected speech, where laryngeal activity must be coordinated with articulatory movement.

Suggestions/Recommendations

At the conclusion of this evaluation, I had the opportunity to share preliminary findings with the team. I will reiterate key points arising in that discussion.

1. Crystal would benefit greatly from a combination of direct and consultative (classroom-based) services. I have enclosed a chapter detailing a treatment program for ataxic dysarthria (authored by Thomas Murry) which should be helpful in generating some specific content during "pull-out" therapy. In light of Crystal's occasional difficulty/shyness adjusting to new people, programming might be carried out by the aide under the supervision/consultation of the speech-language pathologist. The goal should be **functional intelligibility,** with emphasis on enhancing articulatory precision and loudness (these are all interrelated). Work towards increasing intelligibility, concurrent with production of increasingly lengthy chains of syllables in meaningful utterances. Practice/drills involving contrastive stress would also be helpful here, as would pacing (i.e., having her tap concurrent with producing each word or even syllables of words). Employ exaggerated contacts (hard articulatory contacts) in conjunction with drills requiring rapid alternating movements of the articulators.

2. Provide consultation to the classroom teacher relative to expectations of Crystal in the classroom, methods of creating opportunities for successfull interactions with Crystal, correction and modeling procedures, and documentation.[6,11] An example reviewed on the day of my consultation involved calling on Crystal during calendar, asking her the month, then monitoring not only the correctness but also whether or not her answer "March" involved production of the final consonant. Similarly, when she recites the day of the week, the teacher could monitor whether Crystal supplies final consonants and does not delete syllables. This should not be a focus, where Crystal's speech is now in the spotlight—instead the teacher might correct by modeling the correct production, calling on other children (alone or as a group) to repeat the correct production, and so forth.

3. Address phonological processes (directly and consultatively). The use of a minimal contrast program would be appropriate here. Additional opportunities to generalize gains into the classroom can be identified through consultation between the speech-language pathologist and the teacher.

4. The Assessment of Intelligibility of Speech can be readministered, over time, in order to probe changes in intelligibility.

5. With increased attention, Crystal should make significant gains with respect to intelligibility. While her speech may continue to contain multiple misarticulations, I do feel that she has the potential to communicate effectively with all types of listeners across various situations. Augmentative communication does not appear to be warranted at this time.

6. Please feel free to contact me if I can be of any further assistance.

Stephen N. Calculator, Ph.D., CCC-Sp.
Consulting Speech-Language Pathologist

■ APPENDIX D

■ SAM

Speech-Language Consultation

Background Information

Sam was seen for a communication consultation at the High School, where he is a student in the Collaborative Learning

Center. Sam was referred by his classroom teacher, Tom, for assistance with communication programming. Staff have made attempts to integrate students with disabilities into regular classes, yet have never before managed a child with Sam's severity and diversity of needs. At this time, the team sought specific recommendations as to how to enhance Sam's communication skills through the use of augmentative communication techniques and related technology.

Results of psychological testing conducted in May, 1990 indicated intellectual and adaptive skills consistent with the profound range of mental retardation. Sam is blind, nonambulatory (though classified as displaying quadraplegia, his legs are effected significantly moreso than his arms) and nonspeaking. He is highly dependent on staff and others in most activities of daily living, although progress has been noted with respect to his ability to feed himself (with assistance). Communication skills measured by the Vineland Adaptive Behavior Scales were in the 5-12 month range. Results on the Scales of Independent Behavior revealed Social and Communication abilities associated with the 3 month level, developmentally.

The psychologist recommended that Sam's educational program should emphasize functional skills which will prepare him to function in integrated community settings. Communication training was recommended, with a focus on functional skills such as choice making, indicating preferences, and controlling his environment. Relative to the latter, training in switch usage was suggested.

A further review of his record indicates that Sam received consultation from New Hampshire Educational Services for the Sensory Impaired (NHESSI) during the '88-89 school year. At that time he was a student in the Program at the Elementary School. Sam was reportedly able to use a mercury switch which was attached to his forehead using a bandana headband, to activate a tape player. Recommendations following an Occupational Therapy Evaluation included the use of switches to activate age-appropriate leisure time devices and to participate in other meaningful activities.

A comprehensive summary of Sam's medical history can be found elsewhere in his file and will thus not be reiterated here. The most recent speech-language evaluation was conducted in January, 1988. Findings were obtained through parental interview in Sam's home. According to his parents, Sam expresses basic likes and dislikes (e.g., for food) by slapping his hand when happy and screaming when sad or upset. They also reported a discriminate cry to signal his desire for more of a pleasurable activity. Sam reportedly used several words, "Daddy," "Mom," "thank you," "quit that," "bath," and "I eat." He undertood some directions, "raise your arms," when embedded in familiar action sequences/routines.

Present Findings

The present evaluation consisted of observing Sam one morning at school. Observations were supplemented by interviewing team members, and various informal assessment tasks which were introduced concurrent with ongoing instruction in which he was engaged.[12] Impressions were then shared with several team members at the end of the day in order to validate these observations.[1]

After spending a few minutes with Sam, it is understandable why his teacher and others have such a strong, genuine interest in assisting him. Sam is an attractive young man who is highly cooperative. He has a pleasant disposition and is not easily frustrated. Sam deals with change nicely, and does not appear overly disconcerted by shifts in his routines.

Expressively, Sam relies heavily on others to recognize, interpret and then respond to his subtle communicative attempts. He vocalizes frequently, yet these utterances do not appear to convey meaning other than reflecting his concurrent emotional state. For example, the utterance "mamama" was noted by staff (and then observed) to convey Sam was upset. "Daddy" was associated with his being happy and content with a particular activity. His teacher also indicated that this vocalization often occurs in response to Steven's hearing male voices. It was my impression that these vocalizations were used in response to his emotional state at the time and were not used purposefully, nor intentionally, as a way of consciously attempting to effect the actions of others.[14,15]

Upon thinking that he had finished his meal, Sam clasped his hands together at midline and sat patiently. Upon being reoriented to his plate, and finding some additional french fries, he resumed finger feeding. After finding no more food, he again clasped his hands. This behavior appeared to signal that he was done. It was not accompanied by any request for adult attention (such requests were not observed at any time during the obsrvation), nor was it directed to any particular individual. Similarly, he indicated (again perhaps unintentionally) he was finished drinking by releasing his grasp on a cup.[14,15]

While strolling with Sam outdoors, the Aide was asked to suddenly stop and wait for a signal from Sam to resume pushing him.[16] Again, there was no such signal from Sam. He was found to rock his head back and forth as the activity resumed, and then diminished this activity once the chair was again halted. Similar responses were noted when food was presented and then withdrawn from his reach, when he was taken to the threshold of a room and not further, etc.[16] Once again, the behavior (rocking his head from side to side) appeared more a reflection of his emotional state than a conscious attempt to influence others.[15]

Sam did not show any clear means of protesting when his food was removed. On another occasion, food was tapped to his hand and then removed several inches. This did not result in any search behavior on Sam's part. Conversely, upon returning the plate to its predicted location, Sam continued eating. Upon placing a napkin where he expected to find his food, Sam picked up the napkin and started to eat it. He did not appear to respond differentially to this item, not detecting what it was (and was not) despite its familiar feel and predictable presence at meal time.[16]

Sam's behavior varied depending upon with whom he was interacting. He appeared to derive great satisfaction interacting with Mike, as indicated by his smiling, calming, orienting to Mike's voice, and vocalizing.

Staff reported that Sam enjoys being interacted with in a calm and supportive tone of voice, and enjoys being touched (e.g., having his hand stroked as he is interacted with).[6]

Receptively, there is no indication that Sam derives meaning from the content of other's speech. Instead, he has adapted a "do what I would normally do" strategy in responding to predictable commands.[6] For example, when asked to raise his arms so that staff could remove his lap tray, he quickly complied. The extent to which he understood the command, vs. the need to comply given the context (it was time for nap, staff were positioned in a particular location in a predictable location at a particular time of the day) could not be determined.[15]

In summary, Sam's communication needs remain great at this time. In light of the severity of his intellectual disability, deficits in communication are for the most part as expected.[17] Still, there are several modifications to his program which I can suggest at this time, These suggestions build upon Sam's apparent enjoyment being around others and need for nurturance.

Suggestions/Recommendations

1. Staff should be commended for recognizing Sam's needs to be around peers without disabilities. This is an area which should be expanded significantly in the immediate future—moving Sam away from the Learning Center and its affiliated programs and instead into regular classes with appropriate levels of support. The District has applied to participate in the Statewide Systems Change Project next year—this is an excellent first step. The process of change is as exciting as it may, at times, be difficult. In the interim, informal consulation may be arranged to help the team begin identifying additional opportunities and strategies for including Sam in the High School more actively.[2,7,8]

2. It is critical that there be specific instructional expectations of Sam as he moves from class to class. I have attached some materials which should be useful to the team in targeting specific communication and other objectives in various activities. This requires planning between regular and special education (what objectives will be addressed by whom, when; classroom and curriculum modifications; means of measuring progress) and training of the program implementer (e.g., in many cases this might be the Aide).[3]

3. It is critical that staff convey respect for Sam, while also serving as models (for teachers and students) of how to interact appropriately with him. Speak to him as you would another 17 year old. Avoid talking about him in his presence, or ask his permission prior to doing so.[6]

4. Refer to NHATEC for a switch evaluation and information pertaining to how to adapt toys/games, common appliances, etc. Having identified an optimal switch, opportunities to **use it** to access previously unavailable items is essential. Integrate such training with leisure (e.g., music), domestic (e.g., snack preparation—for instance, activating a blender), and other program aspects.

5. The Aide and others should receive training (e.g., from Tom) in the use of Partial Participation and Backward Chaining as methods of enhancing Sam's active participation and independence in everyday activities. For example, at meal time this might take forms such as:

■ Have Sam pay for his own lunch, responding to the cashier's request for money by offering payment.

■ Have Sam select what he wants to eat (e.g., handing the server a note on which his choices have been written out).

In shop class, he might:

■ Indicate which of two tasks he would like to do (present him with an object associated with each, then withdraw. Have Sam reach for the object corresponding to the activity which he desires. Again, given no response, prompt him [up to a full physical prompt] to make a selection.

■ Indicate when he has completed a task [push the completed project aside]. Substitute functionally equivalent responses for behaviors he now uses (e.g., returning to meal time, chain the desired behavior—pushing his tray away, on to the present behavior—clasping his hands.[3]

6. Introduce an object calendar (anticipation shelf) as a means of helping to instill order in Sam's day. Upon arriving, Sam will handle each object (placed in a series of boxes) that corresponds with the day's events.

He will then retreive the first item, which will cue him to report to the first activity. Upon finishing the activity, he will return to the 'calendar' and deposit the object in a "finished box," then retrieve the next object, and so forth.[11]

7. Systematically provide opportunities for choice making throughout the day, using the Activity Planning Matrix. Begin with a high priority, high preference item paired with a neutral or irrelevant object. For example, give him the opportunity to decide whether he wants to take a rest, presenting him with a pillow vs. a bolt. Bring each item to each hand, then withdraw just out of his reach. Ask him which he would prefer to do and then, if necessary, encourage him to reach for the appropriate object (in this case to indicate he wants to take a rest). Gradually, move towards 2 relevant, priority choices and give Sam opportunities to indicate preferences.[3]

8. Consider contracting with a speech-language pathologist who is experienced working with children with Sam's needs, to provide consultation as needed to the school speech therapist. This is particularly necessary in order to get the program up and going, identifying means of measuring progress, modeling for staff, and ongoing program modification. NHESSI can provide information about a statewide system of consultants.[2]

9. Please feel free to call me if I can be of assistance in clarifying the above recommendations.

Sincerely,

Stephen N. Calculator, Ph.D., CCC-Sp.
Consulting Speech-Language Pathologist

■□ APPENDIX E

■□ IVAN

Speech-Language Consultation

Background Information

Ivan was referred by his educational team for a communication consultation. The team sought specific suggestions as to how to proceed with communication programming. Presently, Ivan attends AM Kindergarten at Children's Rainbow then goes on to an afternoon Pre-School/Kindergarten program at the Elementary School. Speech-Language services are provided in the afternoon by Diane, SLP who integrates communication instruction into daily classroom activities.

Ivan was seen for a communication assessment by Janet, SLP at the Communication Center on September 21, 1990. The reader is referred to the resulting report for a description of background information and assessment results. Ivan was felt to be a strong candidate for augmentative and alternative communication. She suggested that staff develop a series of situation-specific mini-boards which contained vocabulary (symbols) specific to ongoing activities. In addition, access to speech output was considered a priority. The use of a computer with speech output and additional software was recommended as a precursor to introducing an electronic communication aid such as the Wolf.

A subsequent speech-language evaluation by Diane revealed findings consistent with that of Janet. Again, it was recommended that Ivan continue to receive speech-language services which emphasized multiple communication modes: pictures, signs, gestures, and vocalizations.

Assessment Procedures and Results

The present assessment consisted of a combination of informal procedures. Ivan was observed at Children's Rainbow (3 hours), then again at the elementary school (2.5 hrs). The examiner was particularly interested in identifying Ivan's present means of communicating and its effectiveness in meeting classroom and related demands.[3,5,12,14] Observations were supplemented by interviews of staff, and sabotage/modifications in routine activities. Results presented below represent the amalgam of skills displayed by Ivan in these two settings.

Ivan quickly impresses others by his friendly, social disposition. He smiles continuously, laughs often, and reinforces others' social advances. The vast majority of his initiations are directed to adults at this time, familiar as well as unfamiliar (such as myself). Initiations most often take the form of direct requests for actions (wants to go out to the playground) and material goods (a doll; a mat; a record player).

According to his teacher at Children's Rainbow, Laura, and his personal Aide, Nan, Ivan does not show signs of being frustrated by an inability to communicate. Both felt that he is quite capable of expressing wants and needs and having these complied with. In observing Ivan, these impressions were quickly validated. Ivan shifts effortlessly and naturally from one communication mode to another, depending on the content of his mesage and his listener's understanding. The same content (a desire to go out and play) was expressed to the same and different listeners, on various occassions, by (1) signing play; (2) pointing to a symbol on his Intro Talker; (3) Taking an adult's hand and pulling them towards the window; (4) Pointing outside.[14]

As indicated above, Ivan rarely engages in meaningful interactions with peers. Typically, peer interactions are limited to touching and gently stroking other children without exchanging additional information.[14] The children at Children's Rainbow were accepting of Ivan and understood his communication limitations. Several of the children used sign with him and all appeared to understand his need to move on from one activity to another rather than engage in prolonged interactions in any given area.[6]

Ivan had a good understanding of his class schedule and often anticipated upcoming events. For example, midway through one activity he would indicate what would be coming up next (e.g., Pointed to 'table' to connote it was time to do some seat work; signed 'music' to connote it was time for free play). Vocalizations were abundant, frequently uttered with a whining intonation. Usually, these consisted of monosyllabic, unintelligible utterances. Vocalizations ceased, temporarily, upon his initial engagement in each successive activity, then quickly resumed. No consistent yes/no response was observed.[14]

Receptively, Ivan's understanding appears to be tied to the contexts in which verbal exchanges occur. It is questionable how much information Ivan receives from the words themselves as opposed to the situation occurring at that particular moment. Ivan effectively employs a strategy of "do what you normally do" when given requests and directions. He seems to tune into a single key word, then predicts what is expected of him based on what he might normally do in a similar situation. Thus when a request is made for him to give an object, while he has a different object already in his possession, his typical response is to offer the object which he is already holding. Ivan had difficulty (or, perhaps refused to comply) with requests that he point to familiar objects when more than one choice was available. Similarly, he responded at a chance level to requests that he give objects based on defining attributes (e.g., the red one, the blue one, the big one, the little one).[14] Comprehension is aided greatly when speech is accompanied by gestures/signs (e.g., pointing towards the location you wish him to go to or to the object you would like him to get).[6] Ivan gives and takes objects on request, when such requests are accompanied by gesture (i.e., reaching towards him or offering him something in one's possession).

Despite the lengthiness of these observations, the examiner is still uncomfortable in saying with certainty that these observations reflect Ivan's competencies, rather than his actual performance. As noted above, Ivan's attention is fleeting much of the time. Often, he no sooner arrives at one activity then he is looking forward to another. Having indicated a desire to visit the babies downstairs at the Children's Rainbow, then asked to indicate this desire on his Intro Talker, he pointed indiscriminately. Similar responses were observed when he used his communication displays. Conversely, when the need was more urgent, and initiated by him, pointing was both purposeful and effective (e.g., to request a turn during circle time).

Recommendations

1. Continue to emphasize a Total Communication approach with Ivan (gestures, signs, vocalizations, pointing, manipulation of objects, communication boards, electronic communication aids). Access to a wide variety of communication modes will continue to increase his liklihood of communication success across various settings, with different listeners, in various activities. No one mode is preferable to another—the preferred mode is that which, in a particular situation, best (and most efficiently) enables Ivan to convey his thoughts and feelings at a given time.

2. Language-based instruction will be of great value to Ivan. It is critical that we remember that in order for him to communicate more effectively, he must have a base of language comprehension skills related to vocabulary (content), syntax (form) and how these skills are employed to satisfy specific purposes (use). Whole language and process oriented aproaches are of great value here. Being exposed to language and concepts in a variety of settings, within themes, will reinforce meaning for him. I have enclosed a catalogue which includes language training activities that can be used with Ivan and the rest of the class. These activities (e.g., Life Experiences Communication Kit and Holiday Kit) promote the use of picture communication symbols within the context of broader language lessons.[11]

Similarly, when interacting with Ivan, it is important that speakers (particularly teachers) modify their verbal input to facilitate comprehension and subsequent development of language. Reduced utterance lengths, increased redundancy, immediate centered content, reduced speaking rate, use of accompanying gestures, etc. are all appropriate at this time. Most importantly, Ivan will thrive in settings in which listeners are highly responsive to him, continuously reinforcing his communication attempts while modeling more elaborate forms, content and uses of language.[6]

3. Communication modes presented to Ivan must have one thing in common—all must have the potential for providing immediate gratification of Ivan's wants and needs. The system must be available at the time the message is being sent. As the latency increases (e.g.,while the system is retrieved from another room or Ivan is removed from the setting in which the need arose and is taken to his communication aid), Ivan's motivation to use the device diminishes accordingly. For this reason, unaided modes of communication continue to offer the greatest flexibility for Ivan.

Staff are encouraged to model gestures/signs when interacting with Ivan and his classmates.[3]

Amer-Ind (American Indian Hand Talk) gestures would be highly functional at this time. These gestures incorporate some signs with which Ivan is already familiar. In addition, these gestures (unlike ASL and SEE) are highly transparent (e.g., guessable) to naive listeners and easily trained. Gestures should be modeled and reinforced in the context of meaningful activities, as indicated above.

4. In those situations in which Ivan is 'contained' (e.g., snack, lunch, circle, table activities) access to miniboards is warranted. All vocabulary available should be relevant to the setting at hand. I have enclosed information regarding how to set up such a system. The use of a Fitzgerald Key (Who, What Doing, What, Where, When, In What Manner) is suggested. Picture Communication Symbols (Don Johnson, Inc.) includes examples of how these categories are employed.[3]

The enclosed catalogue offers alternative methods of displaying symbols as well. Ivan's parents and the rest of the team could identify a system which would be most portable, flexible, with maximum opportunities for expansion over time. The Long Wallet (pg. 27) or Mid-sized Communication Book (pg. 26) are possibilities, both retailing for under $10.00.

5. Access to speech output appears to be a priority of the team, based on our conversations in the past. The use of miniboards, in context, will continue to expose Ivan to the power of communication while prompting continued growth of vocabulary. The same symbols and vocabulary which appear on miniboards can be used on an AAC electronic device.[3]

The Intro Talker is a nice start, however there are limitations relative to the amount of content which can be depicted. Also, the speech is difficult to hear in the noisy background of his classroom. The NHESSI consultant (or PRC Consultant) can furnish information about how this and other devices can be outfitted with an external speaker to increase their loudness. Also relative to the Intro Talker, consider re-programming the aid using a male voice (a boy of a comparable age), rather than his mother's voice.

With certain specifications in mind (ease of programming, flexibility, digitized (rather than synthesized) speech, ease of depicting symbols, my inclination would be to recommend a Small All-Talk, rather than the Intro Talker or Touch Talker. The power of the Touch Talker rests with the user's ability to attach different meanings based not only on the symbols themselves, but the sequences and themes in which they are used. With an All Talk, different overlays could contain different themes, with overlays changing at different times of the day. Each overlay could contain anwhere from 1 to 128 symbols, each containing messages of different durations. Again, the team should consider borrowing this device from NHESSI.

6. As plans are made to transition Ivan to subsequent programs (e.g., Kindergarten, 1st Grade . . .), access to expertise in the area of AAC will continue to be essential. Effective and useful consultation should be available to school staff, emphasizing means of maximizing Ivan's communicative effectiveness in the context of school and outside activities. NHESSI, and NHATEC, both maintain lists of consultants who might be available to assist with Ivan's educational programming.

7. The Team must make every effort to continue to function as such. Where outside assessments are deemed valuable by the team, consensus should be reached as to exactly what information is necessary. Otherwise, we run the risk of continual start-ups as the direction of the program shifts repeatedly. The COACH (Cayuga-Onondaga Assessment for Children with Handicaps, Version 6.0) offers a means of promoting increased collaboration between school and home in setting priorities. Susan has recently received instruction in how to administer this procedure.

8. Please feel free to contact me if I can be of any further assistance. I am convinced that Ivan is in very good hands!

Stephen N. Calculator, Ph.D., CCC-Sp.
Consulting Speech-Language Pathologist

◾ APPENDIX F

◾ ANN

Speech-Langauge Evaluation

Background Information

Ann was referred by Kim, speech-language pathologist for the Elementary Schools, and Marla, Ann's full-time Aide, for a comprehensive communication assessment. The results were to be included in her three year update. In addition, the team was looking for an outside opinion regarding the appropriateness of her present program, and suggestions for how to improve this program.

Marla recounted some of the many significant events which have transpired during her 7 year relationship with Ann. While Ann lives with her grandparents, she spends a majority of her waking hours in Marla's company. She is dropped off at Marla's home at 6:30, Monday through Saturday, and then returns home at 4 PM each day. This schedule is in effect 12 months per year, with additional contact provided during the Summer (e.g., Marla and Ann vacation together).

It became apparent very quickly that Marla's relationship with Ann extends far beyond Aide-Client. There is a strong attachment and mutual respect between the two. Throughout my visit, I was struck by the spontaneity of their interactions, and Marla's commitment to ensure Ann as normal a life style as possible by involving her in the community, neighborhood school, and elsewhere. Marla serves as a primary source of support and security for Ann. Over a 6 hour observation period, Ann continuously displayed a pattern of venturing out to explore new and familiar situations, then returning to Marla's side. She constantly initiated physical interaction with Marla, seeking her out for a quick hug or kiss and then going off on her own. When left alone for brief periods of time with me and/or Kim, Ann showed no signs of protest or upset. Upon Marla's return, Ann quickly reinitiated contact with her.

According to Marla, Ann has improved dramatically over time with respect to decreasing her reliance upon her. In the past, Ann would not allow Marla to leave her alone or in others' company, protesting to the point that Marla was asked (by school personnel) to accompany Ann at all times.

Ann presently attends Wentworth School part-time. She is mainstreamed in a regular fourth grade classroom. In addition, she has a "job" washing trays after lunch in the school cafeteria, goes to the school library, and other locations around the school. The majority of her educational program is provided directly by Marla, within her home. Here, the focus is on goals related to self-management, community, and domestic skills (e.g., doing dishes, washing, drying, and folding laundry, shopping, going to McDonalds, visiting different stores in the community, etc.).

Speech-language consultation is provided by Kim (to Marla) 1x/wk for 30–45 minutes. Consultation consists primarily of sharing ideas as to how to promote choice making, increasing opportunities for communication, ways of restructuring the environment to create needs for communication, etc.

In reviewing the background information which I had access to, there was no evidence of a prior diagnosis of Ann's problems. A psychologic evaluation was recently initiated by the School Psychologist, as part of her three year update. Testing to this point has consisted of administering the Vineland Adaptive Behavior Scales to Judy (the grandmother), Heidi (Ann's fourth grade teacher), and Marla. Preliminary results indicate particularly significant problems in the areas of communication and socialization (age equivalents fall in the 12 to 18 month range), with relative strengths noted in the motor and daily living skills domains (around the three year level). Severe developmental delays were reported across all domains sampled.

Present Assessment

The present assessment consisted of lengthy observations of Ann in natural interactions with familiar adults and peers at Marla's home, and in various locations at school (cafeteria kitchen, library, Mrs. Potter's fourth grade science class; hallways; main office). Observations were supplemented with interviews of Marla and other program providers. In addition, I introduced various informal tasks (myself and/or with Marla's assistance) during ongoing events.

Ann continues to rely on a variety of communication modes to convey her most basic wants and needs. These include the following:

Signs and sign approximations: Signs observed during my visit consisted of "help," "more," and "hi." In addition, she readily imitated signs modeled by Marla (go, start) but failed to use these same signs unless verbally and/or gesturally prompted. Signs were often produced in a distorted manner- particularly with respect to hand orientation and hand shape. Such errors were easily corrected by Marla. According to Marla, Ann rarely signs spontaneously, although she occasionally signs "more" to request more food and to indicate her desire that Marla continue reading to her. She also indicated that Ann's grandparents have not been motivated to sign with her, or to reinforce Ann's signs. Still, she has provided them with resources (e.g., signing dictionaries) and updates of newly introduced signs.

Act on objects: This remains a primary mode of communication for Ann. She spontaneously reaches for and acts upon objects which she desires. Marla has recently introduced an object board for Ann. Actual containers of familiar foods from McDonalds are attached (with velcro) to a cardboard base. Marla reports moderate success having Ann indicate these objects to request corresponding items off the menu at McDonalds.

Proximity seeking: These behaviors appear to serve a social function for Ann. She continuously gravitates back to Marla for hugs and kisses. At other times she positions herself close to Marla, expecting a hug or requesting that she come up on Marla's lap. Over the course of the day, Ann gradually directed some of these same behaviors at me—particularly the proximity seeking. She would stand within a couple of feet of me and appear to study my face. As I moved from pleasant conversation to an attempt to engage her more directly in conversation, she quickly moved off.

Physical manipulation of others: Marla reported that Ann will grab her hand, preventing her from turning off her cassette player in the car, to indicate that she does no want to leave the car and enter a given location.

Vocalizing: No meaningful words are used at this time. Ann was cued to say goodbye—/bu/. She screamed on occasion, not always for any obvious reason. On a few occasions, this behavior was accompanied by signs of physical (though not hurtful) aggression which took the form of grabbing Marla's shirt, neck, and hair. These episodes frequently appeared to be signals that she was simply not happy with what was going on at the time (e.g., being corrected as she washed dishes; being expected to sit idly for extended periods of time as I engaged Marla in conversation, etc. In some instances, there were no obvious antecedents to these outbursts, other than her perhaps being overwhelmed by the events occurring at that given moment.

Yes/No response: Ann nods and shakes her head to indicate yes and no. Yes is also indicated by her complying with requests, acting upon objects offered to her, carrying out requested actions, etc. No is conveyed by refusals to comply, occasional obstinance, ignoring the request (she is very effective in tuning out that which she does not want to hear), and occasional tantrums consisting of screaming and grabbing.

Sensory: Episodes of blowing (sometimes on her listener, other times on her hand, sometimes into open space), breath holding, posturing her hand, fingers, and arm are frequent. These do not appear to serve any function other than they "feel good" to her. They occur in instructional as well as leisure settings, irrespective of whether or not expectations and demands are being placed on her, alone and in the company of others.

Picture pointing: Marla recounted past attempts to develop communication boards and miniboards for Ann. All of these efforts failed due, apparently, to a combined lack of motivation and her inability to use pictures functionally. Informal testing revealed Marla unable to identify a specific object (e.g., a hat) on a page containing multiple stimuli (the hat is on the head of a young boy who is fully dressed and involved in an activity in an even broader context). She employed a strategy of indiscriminately pointing to the most salient feature on the page (e.g., the boy) instead. When directed to focus on two objects (e.g., hat and shoes), she was able to point to one vs. the other on request. Again, this ability varied according to her motivation at any given time.

Marla reported that Ann is very interested in pictures, and greatly enjoys sitting in a chair leafing through a magazine or newspaper. Marla indicated that Ann fixates on a picture for several seconds before continuing to peruse the material.

Ann's comprehension abilities are greatly tied to context at this time. Comprehension is greatly facilitated by using simplified input. Ann seems to tune into a single key word in each utterance directed to her. Where a key word is not embedded in a complex set of instructions or a multi-utterance request she is more likely to respond appropriately. Marla was very adept at simplifying her language to meet Ann's needs. Utterances were simple and often repeated and/or paraphrased. The same meaning would be presented two and three times, with slight variations in her choice of words—a process known as scaffolding.

On numerous occasions, what appeared to be a lack of comprehension was instead found to be a lack of willingness to comply on Ann's part. Ann would stare off in space or withdraw from the interaction. With greater persistence, she then complied with the request being made of her.

Comprehension included topics which were familiar and yet non-immediate. For example, while seated in the living room, she was told "Let's do the wash," resulting in her standing up and making her way to the laundry room. Requests to "wash her hands,""turn on the light" (after already leaving the room in which she was in, thus constituting an improbable request) were responded to correctly. As additional key elements were included (e.g. a desired location, an action, and a set of objects), she performed more erratically. For example, when asked to "Put the book on the table," she placed it on a couch instead. A two part command, "Put it (the laundry) in and close the door" resulted in her performing the latter part of the activity and not the former.

In summary, Ann is a young girl with tremendous needs. She would benefit greatly from communication training which is systematically integrated within a broader educational program. Her Aide, Marla, continues to be a tremendous source of nurturance and instructional support. The following suggestions and recommendations are offered at this time.

Recommendations

1. An examination of Ann's present IEP reveals a lack of educational goals for those times in which she is mainstreamed, isolated delivery of related services, and an apparent lack of prioritization of educational goals. There do not appear to be a set of shared educational goals among the various team members. I would greatly encourage the team to generate an I.E.P. using the C.O.A.C.H. process. Marla would be the likely informant in conducting this process, with additional information secured by Marla's grandparents and others at the team's discretion. I have sent ordering information related to the COACH to Marla and to Paul Andrade. The procedure takes approximately 2 hours to administer and can result in a set of prioritized goals as well as a plan as to how to address educational needs in the context of regular education.

2. Ann should be in an **age**-appropriate placement. Once again, the COACH provides tools for examining curriculum and activities and modifying or substituting alternative activities as appropriate. We do not want to place Ann in a situation in which she is present but not really a part of a class activity. There should be clear expectations of Ann at school, with all concerned aware of the educational goals being addressed at any given time. I have attached a copy of a handout displaying a format by which specific IEP goals can be targeted in regular education settings, and a second format for determing the need to modifiy activities and/ or address different skills than those arising in a particuular classroom. I reviewed both of these forms with Kim Leaman and Marla during my visit and would be happy to review them with other team members as well.

During my visit, I found Kim, Marla, the school librarian and others all very capable of generating alternative curriculum for Ann. For example, a trip to the library resulted in our mini team generating a list of activities which would be beneficial for Ann given the prescribed activity that day was not deemed appropriate or worth modifying. These same activities could constitute school jobs for Ann. They included sorting books ready for reshelving by fiction (red circle) and non-fiction (green circle); working with a peer in signing books out/stamping books; sorting magazines vs. books; reshelving materials by cueing into a call number or letter. We also discussed encouraging Ann to use her name stamp to sign out her own materials, and as a means of providing personal identification (with her signature) throughout the day.

Similarly, science class was seen as providing multiple opportunities for learning new and exciting things in the company of peers. Where the content was over her head, once again a menu of alternative activites within the room should be available. Such activities should reinforce IEP objectives/educational priorities. For example, she might spend some of her time watering the plants, tidying up the room, setting up the experiments by gathering the necessary materials and helping to distribute them to classmates, and so forth.

3. Identify other worthwhile jobs in and around school. Ann's classmates represent a potential source of ideas and problem solving. They could generate alternative activities and goals (e.g., when watering plants, her goal might be to fill up a vase with water to a designated spot on the vase; to turn the faucet on and off; to return the plant to its original location, etc.).

4. Consider identifying an area of the classroom to which Ann can choose to go to collect herself. Before becoming overly agitated (I realize that these episodes often occur with little warning), she might be encouraged to excuse herself from a class activity and have some quiet time. A bean bag chair positioned out of the flow of activity, with a box containing various magazines and books, might be a much needed sanctuary for Ann when things are overly hectic for her.

5. Integrate choice making and request goals (see progress report by Kim) into school and home activities using the Matrix format.

6. Model signs in conjunction with verbal input. Encourage classmates to start using a small repertoire of signs with her as well, giving the impression that sign is an acceptable mode of communication in the classroom. AMERIND (American Indian Hand Talk) may be advantageous to ASL for Ann in that its gestures are highly iconic (gestures are very guessable and look like the objects/actions that they represent, unlike many of the signs in ASL, which are often arbitrary in nature). AMERIND is significantly more intelligible to naive listeners, more easily acquired, and more likely to be retained by Ann and her classmates. A copy of this dictionary is available at the UNH library. (Note: Many of the ASL signs, particularly the highly iconic ones, are similar if not the same as their AMERIND counterparts.)

7. The district should consider contracting with a special education consultant to support this program in the role of integration facilitator. Staff at the Institute on Developmental Disability at UNH, may be of assistance in locating such a person if no one is available in district at this time.

8. Marla and others are encouraged to observe other districts' efforts at integrating children with severe disabilities into regular education. I encourage you to contact the principal at the Robert School. They are doing a beautiful job with a young boy with severe disabilities, incuding many autistic-like behaviors. I feel this would be a good situation to observe in that the Aide assumes primary responsibility for direct instruction, yet receives the support of the classroom teacher and classmates. The principal is a true visionary.

9. The team might consider sponsoring a workshop on inclusive schooling/rationale for integrating children with severe disabilities into regular education. Again, depending on the needs and objectives, I would be happy to suggest the names of possible speakers.

10. Continue to employ a total communication approach with Ann. Try to limit the amount of prompting/cueing, having Ann rely more on her own. For example, she might be cued to stay on task by a sequence of photographs depicting the various stages of a job which she is expected to perform (e.g., the laundry). She could check off under each photograph as she completes each portion of the task.

11. I have attached a copy of an article on object communication boards for Kim and Marla's use. They may pick up some useful suggestions given they feel it worthwhile to pursue training via this mode.

12. Re-evaluate Ann's progress in six months, given the above changes are implemented.

If I can be of any further assistance, please do not hesitate to call. Ann is indeed fortunate to have surrounded herself with such a caring group of friends and professionals. I applaud your efforts.

Stephen N. Calculator, Ph.D., CCC-Sp.
Consulting Speech-Language Pathologist

Footnotes for Appendices A–F

1. Assessment results are nothing more than impressions. They only become findings upon others' confirming their accuracy and relevance.

2. Part of the assessment should include delineating environmental supports. Identify critical adults who will play a role in enhancing communication/participation of the student in daily events.

3. Delineate academic/curricular expectations as a basis for subsequent discrepancy analysis (does the student have the necessary communication skills for participation in an existing, or projected, curriculum)?

4. You Can Only Have a Team Once You Settle on a Field

5. Discrepancy analysis with subsequent focus on intervention which will focus on promoting participation of students in daily events.

6. Assessment may examine others' styles of interaction with the student, examining their appropriateness and usefulness [relative to supporting/enhancing communication and participation].

7. Assess nature of supports, and consider changes in roles which will enhance involvement of classmates (vs. adult centered).

8. Identify present as well as potential opportunities for participation.

9. Assess future communication needs.

10. Review prior communication instruction. Look to the future with an awareness of what has been introduced in the past.

11. Delineate instructional strategies (e.g., teaching modifications)which would enhance students' participation.

12. Assess communication in a variety of natural settings, with a variety of conversational partners.

13. Formal test results must be examined and validated relative to other, informal sources of information.

14. Describe existing means of communication, particularly for students who rely on ambiguous, unconventional means of communication. These behaviors must be described so that others can interpret and respond to students appropriately.

15. Comment on the intentionality of students' behavior, where necessary.

16. Use analogue assessment to supplement natural observations.

17. Examine severity of communication problems relative to other areas of functioning (mental age and intra-linguistic referencing) in order to help determine the extent to which students might benefit from instruction.

Communicative Intervention as a Means to Successful Inclusion

Stephen N. Calculator

■ INTRODUCTION

In Chapter 4, we reviewed a variety of assessment practices that can be used to identify communication skills necessary for students with severe disabilities to effectively participate in regular classrooms. Chapter 5 delineates the role of SLPs *and others* in addressing communication problems and in developing communication strengths. The chapter begins by reviewing some guiding principles for communication intervention. These principles are then operationalized through case studies to illustrate a variety of instructional strategies.

■□ COMMUNICATION AND INCLUSION: CHICKEN OR EGG?

Ferguson (1992) suggests that our goal should not be one of fostering communication, but instead, *membership*. She states, "The purpose of all of our interventions, programs, indeed, schooling in general is to enable all students to actively participate in their communities so that others care enough about what happens to them to look for ways to include them as part of that community" (p. 9). Does more effective communication foster inclusion, or is the relationship between these concepts captured better by a hypothesis stating that inclusion fosters more effective communication?

It is now considered very important to examine factors such as settings, purposes and outcomes of communication when designing instructional programs for students with severe disabilities. We now acknowledge that any interaction proceeds from the shared experiences, goals, desires, wants, and needs of the participants. **Communication is nothing less than an overt expression of interdependence among people.** As such, where there is no interdependence we might not expect communication to arise.

For example, classmates are unlikely to issue requests to a student from whom, based on previous experiences, they do not expect a response. Students are unlikely to relate personal information and feelings to people who fail to reinforce such efforts. There is a personal and/or shared history leading up to any specific communicative exchange.

■□ MAINTAINING THE REGULAR CURRICULUM

Mirenda and Calculator (1993) stress the need to include students with severe disabilities in the regular curriculum to the greatest extent possible. As discussed in Chapter 3, the actual goals for these students are often different from their classmates'. However, the opportunity to learn in the same setting, with similar materials (e.g., worksheets and books) that are used by classmates, promotes opportunities for working together, supporting one another, exchanging comments, and so forth. By modifying the communication requirements of a particular task, students who might otherwise have required alternate programs may now participate in their regular classroom. Mirenda and Calculator point out that these experiences enhance students' perceptions of themselves while showing others that they are able to participate successfully in regular classroom activities.

Conversely, when a student has a personalized curriculum, opportunities for interaction with others may be limited. The student often works alone, or with a personal aide, minimizing interactions with classmates. A signal may be sent to the rest of the class that what they are doing is not relevant to the student.

To implement communicative interventions that foster inclusion, SLPs and others may need to adopt a functional orientation that views communication in the broader contexts of participation and inclusion. Principles that are consistent with this perspective are summarized in Table 5–1.

TABLE 5–1
Guiding principles for communicative intervention

1. Communication instruction is relevant to the extent that it fosters interactions and inclusion.
2. Communication is best viewed as a support (for interaction and inclusion), rather than an independent area of the curriculum.
3. Students communicate for different reasons and purposes.
4. Communication is a means to an end, not an end in itself.
5. Communication must represent a means of enhancing students' independence, rather than their unnecessary dependence on others.
6. All students communicate.
7. There are no prerequisites to communication.
8. No one mode of communication is always preferable to another.
9. Teach communicative behaviors that will be effective with a range of listeners.
10. Avoid replacing one idiosyncratic mode of communication with another.
11. Changes in communication systems can only enhance communication when students participate in classrooms and other settings that foster interaction.
12. Communication should be a tool for interaction and not simply an attractive prop.

■❑ COMMUNICATION INSTRUCTION IS RELEVANT TO THE EXTENT THAT IT FOSTERS INTERACTIONS AND INCLUSION

The student with communication problems is one who is unable to create and respond to communication opportunities at different times of the day, in different settings, and with different people. Chapter 4 described different methods (e.g., discrepancy analyses, analogue assessments, dynamic assessments, and so forth) of elucidating students' individual communicative needs. Chapters 2 and 3 provided information about incorporating communication objectives and goals into the general education curricula. To assess the outcomes of these activities (relative to inclusion), educational personnel and parents might consider examining corresponding changes in students' lives. This subject will be addressed later in this chapter.

■❑ COMMUNICATION IS BEST VIEWED AS A SUPPORT FOR INTERACTION AND INCLUSION, RATHER THAN AN INDEPENDENT AREA OF THE CURRICULUM

It is helpful to view communication as one of many areas in which support(s) might be necessary to enhance inclusion and participation. Jorgensen (1992) defines natural supports as "those components of an educational program-philosophy, policies, people, materials and technology, curricula-which are used to enable all students to be fully participating members of regular classroom, school, and community life. Natural supports bring children closer together as friends and learning partners rather than isolate them" (p. 5).

As our reliance on natural supports increases, the role of professionals should not diminish in significance. Parents may find it disconcerting when it is suggested that their children require less direct contact with an SLP. They may misinterpret this as implying that communication is no longer a priority need of their children. Although this issue is discussed elsewhere in this book, it is important that we address it here as well.

The team that operates as an aggregate of professionals, each with circumscribed areas of expertise, has no difficulty assigning goals to corresponding experts. Needs in the areas of dressing, toileting, manipulation of objects, pointing, and so forth fall in the province of OT. Goals addressing the enhancement of communication (e.g., increasing the frequency with which students intitiate messages, request clarification, use their augmentative devices, and so forth) fall in an SLP's domain. Paperwork is neat and succinct as signatures are placed in discrete areas of one document after another, each of which is passed from person to person at the conclusion of an IEP planning meeting.

Conversely, when viewing communication as a support, roles overlap significantly. Every individual who is in contact with a student is a potential source of support for communication use and enhancement. The SLP plays an instrumental role in working with the team (to include the student, parents, classmates, teachers, and others) in several capacities, as summarized in Table 5–2.

The activities illustrated in Table 5–2 reflect a "least intrusive supports first" orientation (Jorgensen, 1992). When it is determined that a student requires assistance to participate in an activity, that assistance is optimally provided by classmates first and then, if need be, by their general education teachers, aides, and (least optimally) other special educators. The SLP helps to identify the types of support a student needs at different times of the day in order to maximally participate in the general curriculum. Activities carried out by others, in support of inclusion, are reviewed below.

Supports From Classmates

Where the need for supports (in the form of people) is identified, the SLP might begin by considering if classmates might occupy this role. This is no different than situations in which nondisabled students find themselves when confronted with a problem. Students are often encouraged to seek help from one another, to work cooperatively and collaboratively with one another, to seek clarification, missing information, and so forth.

For the student with severe disabilities, it is important that classmates are aware of how this student communicates (similar to and different from methods used by themselves and other classmates). Methods of programming communication aids can also be shared with students.

Classmates who are particularly fond of the student can be observed and, if need be, interviewed (in the student's presence)

TABLE 5–2

Types of communication supports that might be provided by SLPs (and others) to enhance students' inclusion and participation in general education

1. Collaborate with others (particularly the classroom teacher) to identify, implement, and then monitor the impact of classroom and curriculum modifications. These supports are designed to assure that the student's educational needs are being addressed within the regular curriculum.

   a. During art class, a classmate will encourage John to show his completed project to another student.

   b. The classroom aide will review the teacher's lesson plan and then program messages on Laura's communication device to make sure she can offer pertinent content when this activity occurs later in the day.

   c. A classmate will offer Sarah a choice of two books, either of which the peer is prepared to read to her, during silent reading.

   d. The classroom teacher is asked by the SLP to purposely mumble two questions to Paul one day, then record Paul's response. Later the teacher and SLP develop a plan, which incorporates modeling by classmates, to encourage Paul to request clarification and repetition in these and subsequent (actual) situations.

2. Identify communication demands of the curriculum (teacher input, peer input, materials used, responses expected) relative to student's abilities. (Previous chapters have reviewed specific protocol for conducting such analyses).

3. Identify the need for augmentative communication, and develop an appropriate AAC system (e.g., method of depicting symbols, type of output, type of display, means of accessing the system [e.g., choice of switch].

4. Collaborate with others (teachers, parents, classmates) to discern the role of the AAC system, relative to extant modes of communication, in enhancing a student's level of participation in school activities. Reinforce the notion that the AAC system is a means and not an end.

   a. John shines a flashlight on a picture denoting that it is "sunny", in response to his teacher's asking the class, "Can anyone tell me what it is like outside today?"). Later, he uses a smile vs. frown to respond to yes/no questions. Still later, he points to symbols in his communication book to select a classroom job that he would like to perform that day.

   b. Tara's goal of indicating choices at meal time is suspended. Classmates have wondered why she has such an opportunity, whereas they are expected to eat everything sent from home. In addition, all agree that it is more important that she feed herself than rely on others to provide food in response to her requests. Other times in a day's schedule for addressing choice making are determined (e.g., equipment she would like to be taken to during recess, a musical instrument she wishes to play, a classmate with whom she would like to work). These are all choices that are available to other children as well and choices that arise naturally in her existing curriculum.

5. Purchase necessary supplies and equipment.
   a. Several teachers and related service staff are on the mailing lists of major manufacturers.
   b. Catalogs and other pertinent information are shared with teachers, parents, and other team members.
   c. One person is designated to pursue the purchase of a communication device. The helper contacts vendors and arranges for a demonstration of the device at school.

6. Maintain and service supplies and equipment.
   a. A team member is identified who can help teachers and others troubleshoot when a problem is encountered with Jennie's communication device. This same individual assumes responsibility for communicating with the manufacturer.
   b. A classmate removes Phil's communication board from his lap tray and places it in a safe location when a particular activity counterindicates its use.

7. Continuously monitor the student's motivation and attitudes about their communication system.
   a. The teacher maintains a log, for 3 consecutive days, of situations in which a student uses a communication device. The instructor also notes situations in which use of the device would have been warranted, in that it could have led to more effective and efficient communication, but had not been employed.
   b. The SLP maintains ongoing contact with the student, classmates, and others to identify problems/limitations of the communication system, and to brainstorm possible solutions.
   c. The school counselor develops a procedure for monitoring the student's frequency of socially inappropriate/challenging behaviors. Staff have found these behaviors increase in contexts in which the student is unable to express thoughts and feelings with her present communication system.

8. Collaborate with classroom teacher and aide to identify changes in instructional style and philosophy that can promote increased interaction among students (e.g., cooperative learning).

9. Home-school coordination.
   a. Highlights of the school day are briefly summarized in a notebook that goes home with the student (and is returned, with similar information, from home back to school). The communica-

TABLE 5–2
(continued)

---

tion system provides a means by which Tom can answer
questions and provide additional novel information about topics
that are briefly alluded to in the notebook.

10. Appropriate and effective methods of interacting with the student
are modeled for others. The student takes as active a role in the
training of listeners as possible.

   a. Jamal has a recorded message on his augmentative device that
politely asks his listener to refrain from interrupting him.

   b. Sheila's communication notebook includes a brief description of
her system and some tips on how others can use it with her
effectively. She directs both unfamiliar and familiar persons to
these instructions.

---

to determine their strategies for effectively conversing with the
student. This can occur as part of a larger conversation involving
the entire class. Students can discuss what they feel to be social-
communicative attributes of people with whom they enjoy conversing, as opposed to those associated with people whom they try
to avoid.

At the same time, difficulties can be expressed (messages they
wish the student could convey, need for clearer indications that
the student understands them, and so forth). A plan for addressing classmates' concerns could be engineered by the SLP (in collaboration with others).

Support From Teachers and Aides

Continuing with this "least intrusive supports first" orientation, the
SLP might next consider enlisting support from classroom teachers and aides/paraprofessionals. The results of a communication
assessment can help to identify optimal ways of interacting with
a particular student. For example, a teacher may refer to pictures on
a student's communication board as he lectures about a related topic.

Some students may be more likely to participate in classes in
which their teachers simplify their language, accompany speech
with signs and gestures, and incorporate students' communication
systems into their lessons. It is important that teachers simplify their
language to correspond with a student's level of comprehension.

Such adaptations can also be accomplished by a classmate's paraphrasing instructions for the student.

On other occassions (e.g., story hour), the teacher might be encouraged to read "normally." The oral language might be manageable for the student (given the support of corresponding pictures that accompany the text). Regardless, story hour is a context that encourages social interaction, role play, question-answer, and so on. Any of these activities may be of greater significance than the particular details of the story being read.

The school SLP can collaborate with teachers and others to delineate the communication expectations associated with classroom activities and events, then develop a plan for providing instructional supports for particular students. We have found the Teacher Skill Checklist (McGinnis & Goldstein, 1984) to be useful for assessing skills deemed essential for students' succcess in classrooms. A rater who is familiar with the student responds to 60 questions, which can be classified into five areas: (a) classroom survival skills (e.g., Does the student remember the books and materials needed for class?); (b) friendship-making skills (e.g., Does the student know how and when to begin a conversation with another person?); (c) skills for dealing with feelings (e.g., Does the student identify feelings he or she is experiencing?); (d) skill alternatives to aggression (e.g., Does the student accept losing at a game or activity without becoming upset or angry?); (e) skills for dealing with stress (e.g., Is the student able to relax when tense or upset?). Behaviors are rated on a Likert-type scale (1–5) that guages the relative presence of positive social skills. The SLP and other team members can then prioritize problems identified on the Checklist, and propose strategies for teaching necessary skills to the student.

Support From Special Education Teachers

Assistance (on the continuum of "least intrusive supports") might next be sought from special education teachers/consultants or as they are sometimes referred to, integration/inclusion coordinators. Locke and Mirenda (1992) published the results of a national (USA) survey of more than 200 special education teachers who served on teams that provided AAC supports to students. The investigators were particularly interested in determining the types of roles and responsibilities these educators served.

Most of the respondents had a master's degree, had received some formal training in AAC, and were assisting 6 to 10 students with AAC needs in public schools. It should be noted that 90% of the respondents worked in self-contained classrooms; fewer than 4% served students primarily in regular classrooms.

Roles acknowledged by greater than 70% of the special educators were: adapting the curriculum (87%); identifying vocabulary to include on the AAC device (84%); preparing and maintaining documentation (83%); writing AAC goals and objectives for the students (82%); assessing cognitive abilities (81%); determining students' motivation and attitudes toward AAC techniques (78%); home-school coordination (75%); determining students' communication needs (77%).

Further questioning by Locke and Mirenda (1992) revealed that these roles were ones that respondents preferred to assume and also felt qualified assuming. SLPs should be particularly alerted to Locke and Mirenda's reporting that only 28% of the teachers indicated that their role included instructing significant others in the use of AAC. Given what we know about the need for information about communication skills and the potential impact of AAC, this is certainly an area that needs to be addressed by SLPs and others.

As Locke and Mirenda indicate, their respondents are not necessarily representative of the larger population of special education teachers, many of whom have received little or no formal training in AAC and/or have limited experience providing AAC supports to students with severe disabilities. However, the results indicate that these professionals can play a highly significant role in supporting students with severe communication needs.

Similarly, it is difficult to extrapolate from the findings a role for special educators who are supporting students in regular education settings. However, it should be pointed out that *students' classmates, regular classroom teachers, aides, and others can occupy these same roles depending on their respective levels of competence and the availability of ongoing support (as needed).*

■⬚ STUDENTS COMMUNICATE FOR DIFFERENT REASONS AND PURPOSES

Returning to Table 5–1, principle three suggests that SLPs, teachers, parents and others should consider students' reasons and purposes for communicating, when designing instructional programs. Students communicate to make requests, indicate wants and needs, comment on events around them, provide novel information, exchange greetings, compliment peers and teachers, and so forth. Communication interventions should thus enhance students' abilities to communicate in these many ways. A student who can label (e.g., by signing or pointing to symbols on a communication display) 20 objects has acquired a skill with few possible applications. However, a classmate who is able to *use* signs and symbols to request objects, to make requests for more, to reject objects, to offer objects to others, to comment on objects, and to call attention to objects is more likely to meet daily communication demands in classrooms and other settings.

Glennen and Calculator (1985) demonstrate that students who are able to use symbols for one purpose (e.g., labeling) may be unable to use these same symbols for other purposes such as requesting. Instruction that targets different uses of symbols may be necessary, rather than assuming that students will automatically generalize their use of symbols to meet different environmental demands.

■ COMMUNICATION IS A MEANS TO AN END, NOT AN END IN ITSELF

Communication has value to the extent that it enables students to connect with people and events around them, and to alter their surroundings as different needs arise. Communication for the student with severe disabilities is not a device, an output or input mode, or a symbol set. These components can enhance students' communication skills by accelerating their rates of communication and expanding the range of topics and ideas about which they communicate. However, while such changes are often necessary they are not sufficient to engender changes in the quality of students' daily interactions with others, as was illustrated to the first author (SC) several years ago by Kevin, who taught me a great deal about what communication is, and what it is not.

> Kevin was 10 years old when SC first met him
> 9 years ago. His primary modes of communication
> *(continued)*

were his warm smile and expressive blue eyes. These gestures were accompanied by a frown, which was easily interpreted. Also, Kevin had a repertoire of coos, squeals, hums, and other vocalizations that conveyed pleasure/displeasure, assent/dissent, and so forth.

In observing Kevin in his classroom, I was struck by the ease with which he communicated with others. Much of this could be credited to his ability to place peers, teachers, and others at ease when interacting. Listeners combined a 20-questions approach with rich interpretation and confirmation of his nonverbal behavior.

As the SLP charged with developing an effective means of communication for Kevin, I began with what was then believed to be a starting point for communication intervention: development of a reliable and conventional yes/no response. A simple speech output device was introduced, and Kevin was encouraged to activate switches to the right and left of his head to trigger recorded yes/no messages.

Next, I targeted Kevin's disproportionately strong reliance on others to select and initiate topics of conversation, and his inability to contribute novel information in ensuing conversations. Numerous hours of assessment and intervention culminated in an eye gaze system that I affectionately labeled the Unicolor Binary Visual Encoding Board (UCBVEB).

Through a series of eye gazes, Kevin was able to encode items (pictures) in 64 different locations around a plexiglass board. The UCBVEB procedure required listeners to verbalize where they felt Kevin was looking at on his display, Kevin confirming or rejecting these guesses, then supplying the second coordinate, to convey the location of one of the 64 pictures displayed.

As Kevin's *communication* program proceeded, the quantity and quality of interactions with people other than me appeared to suffer. Unlike his original means of communication, the new technique required increased assistance from listeners. Classmates and teachers now struggled to talk about things that could somehow prompt Kevin to use his communication board. What, if anything, he had to say was suddenly less important than that he used his UCBVEB to say it.

Kevin now had a discrete means of indicating yes/no. He had progressed from unconventional gestures to the use of conventional pictures and line drawings to convey his basic wants and needs. He had even displayed an ability to string two or more pictures together to create novel messages. Yet, these accomplishments had left him more isolated than ever. Frustrations mounted, breakdowns in communication increased, and soon others appeared to be avoiding contact with Kevin.

Kevin was subjected to hours of "therapy" and "instruction" to enhance his communication effectiveness. Teachers and peers were subjected to hours of in-service training on how to communicate with Kevin, how to make him a more active participant in conversations, how to encourage his use of the communication board and speech output aid. Again, net gains seen in therapy appeared be at the expense of natural interactions in and out of the classroom.

Kevin tried to reject this program in many ways: unreliable eye pointing to pictures that everyone knew he understood, refusals to respond, attempts to vocalize and use other natural gestures rather than his new modes, laughing each time the board, having been incorrectly attached to his wheelchair, fell to the ground. The other students in his classroom also expressed their rejection: "I don't need the board, Kevin and I do fine without it." Still the "program" necessitated its use and rationalized any short-term inconveniences that might be experienced by Kevin and others along the way.

(continued)

Attempts (by other SLPs, teachers and others) such as these plagued Kevin for several years. New switches were introduced, methods of depicting messages changed from pictures to line drawings and some words, and the eye gaze was supplemented with a light mounted on top of his head, which Kevin could use to select items on his display, and so forth. However, the most effective method by which Kevin communicated and chose to communicate remained his original set of gestures and vocalizations. Similarly, this remained the method of choice of others when outside the watchful eye of the SLP.

Meanwhile, Kevin's parents never seemed to find the time to learn how to operate the UCBVEB. In fact, they indicated that they were content that this and subsequent systems remained at school. Unlike the "experts" at school, their common sense enabled them to resist programs and *communication props* that would impede interactions with their son.

Kevin's classmates viewed him as a warm and friendly boy with whom they could exchange thoughts and ideas. Topics were not provided by an SLP. Instead, subject matter arose spontaneously and naturally in the context of experiences that were shared by Kevin and his peers. When a classmate related a funny anecdote to Kevin and he smiled, the storyteller's perception of himself as a humorist was supported. When a classmate related a sad occurrence to Kevin and he looked somber, it was often enough to help the former develop a plan to set matters on a more positive course.

So long as the classroom context supported opportunities in which Kevin and others had shared experiences, communication was a natural concomitant. However, problems arose when communication (rather than interaction) became a target for instruction.

A second example of mistakenly targeting communication as an end rather than a means was demonstrated with Toni. Her teachers and SLP had determined that Toni needed to initiate messages more often. They reasoned that it would be helpful (to

Toni) if she was required to make requests as often as possible throughout the day. However, rather than pairing such requests with functional activities and valued consequences, the following program was implemented.

Classmates of Toni were expected to store their books and materials in their desks, to return materials to their appropriate location, and to maintain an orderly work area. If their teacher asked them to complete an assignment, they were expected to quietly gather any materials that would be necessary for them to comply. Conversely, Toni found herself in a "communication" program in which her Aide purposely sabotaged her environment by hiding and purposely misplacing Toni's materials. Toni was then prompted to use her communication book to request (from her aide) the materials that she needed to comply with her teacher's requests. Not unexpectedly, Toni often shifted her attention to other activities occurring in the classroom, as her aide attempted to bring her back "on task." Rather than serving the intended purpose of fostering opportunities for Toni to communicate, these activities instead prompted Toni to seek interaction elsewhere.

■ COMMUNICATION MUST REPRESENT A MEANS OF ENHANCING STUDENTS' INDEPENDENCE RATHER THAN THEIR UNNECESSARY DEPENDENCE ON OTHERS

Unlike Toni, we have observed students who have been encouraged to organize their desks and work areas, and to independently (without communicating) select materials they felt were necessary to comply with their teachers' directions. Communication (in these types of tasks) only became appropriate when these students needed materials such as scissors, knives, paints, musical instruments, water, paper, and staplers that required their teachers' permission and/or assistance. These same situations would have represented appropriate opportunities for communication instruction for Toni.

■□ ALL STUDENTS COMMUNICATE

In Chapter 4, procedures for identifying students' existing methods of communication were described. We operate under an assumption that all students communicate, some more effectively than others. As diagnosticians, our role includes determining the ways and corresponding effectiveness that students interact with others. Instruction generally builds on students' existing methods of communication, rather than replacing socially appropriate behaviors that are already serving some of the student's needs. Our focus, in communication instruction, must be on those situations in which students' existing communication repertoires are proving to be insufficient for interaction and participation in inclusive classrooms.

■□ THERE ARE NO PREREQUISITES TO COMMUNICATION

If we accept the notion that all students communicate, we should never find ourselves teaching communication prerequisites. In the past, students were not felt to be *ready* for communication until they showed evidence of possessing certain cognitive skills, such as an understanding of object permanence, causality, means-ends, imitation, symbolic play, and so forth. More recently, investigators (Kangas & Lloyd, 1988; Reichle, Feeley & Johnston, 1993; Reichle & Karlan, 1985) have rejected this notion of cognitive prerequisites and have instead suggested employing zero exclusion criteria to identify students who might benefit from communication instruction.

Shelley provides an example of educators delaying communication instruction in favor of teaching cognitive prerequisites. A more appropriate way of addressing cognition and communication together, as part of a broader focus on interaction, participation, and inclusion, is also illustrated in this case study.

I (SC) arrived in Shelley's preschool classroom and found her working with an aide in the back of the room. A plate switch attached to a battery operated toy was positioned in the center of a table. When Shelley hit the switch, cookies would bounce around (always for 5 seconds) inside a container presided over by Cookie Monster.

The aide instructed Shelley to hit the switch, then gave her 5 seconds to comply. "Correct" responses were "naturally" reinforced (i.e., cookies were set in motion). Failures to respond resulted in the aide offering Shelley hand-over-hand assistance to activate the switch.

In reviewing data gathered over a period of months, Shelley's performance appeared erratic. Her aide interpreted this to indicate the need for ongoing training. She suggested that Shelley failed to consistently grasp the underlying notion of means (the switch) ends (toy activation) behavior.

Additional observations of Shelley revealed frequently unsuccessful attempts to engage others in interaction. Shelley was usually positioned on the floor, with several toys within her reach. Other children and adults walked past but rarely approached her. As others entered her sight, Shelley often looked at and smiled in their direction, but for naught. These behaviors routinely went unnoticed. Interviews with other children and adults indicated that they did not feel Shelley was aware that they existed.

Shelley was provided with a switch (the same one that she had used inconsistently to activate Cookie Monster), yet this time it was attached to a tape recorder. When Shelley hit the switch, a recorded message ("Hi, can you come over and talk awhile?") played repeatedly until the switch was released. Not only did Shelley quickly learn to activate the switch, but she also learned to use this action (*as a means*) to initiate interactions with others (*an ends*).

Prerequisites and Bedknobs

Shelley's program illustrated a case in which a nonfunctional "communication" goal, in this case a perceived cognitive prerequisite, was successfully replaced by an activity with immediate and functional consequences for her and those around her. When will we stop wasting valuable time teaching prerequisites to behaviors that are already in evidence in the communication repertoires of our students? Mary, another student, must have asked this question on numerous occasions.

Mary's program encouraged improved visual tracking skills. Each day, Mary was sat down and prompted to follow lights and other objects that were introduced along various horizontal and vertical axes. How puzzling it must have all seemed to Mary. Didn't anyone notice that each time there was a visitor to the classroom, she looked at the individual and then tracked the latter's movements around the room?

I recall carrying Mary out of her living room at home and noticing that as we traversed the room she maintained eye contact with an illuminated aquarium located in a distant corner. Later that visit, while talking with her mother, I noticed Mary struggling to lift her head from the floor. She was lying on her stomach over a bolster in front of the television. Mary would raise up her head for as long as 5 seconds to watch "Sesame Street," then drop her head to the floor. While her head was raised, her eyes followed the images on the television screen.

Mary's physical therapist (PT) questioned the validity of my observations, just as she had listened politely to similar reports over the years from Mary's mother. The reaction was not exceptionally unusual, given Haring's (1988) finding that **21% of the skills being taught to students with severe disabilities by their experienced teachers had been already**

acquired. One of Mary's goals at school required her to raise her head, from the prone position and maintain it in an upright position for 3 seconds. The therapist noted that Mary's performance of this skill had been erratic the past year. Clearly, **the likelihood that skills will be demonstrated by *all* students depends as much on the nature of the task as it does on their actual abilities**.

In the case of Mary, the team agreed that throughout the day, teachers and others should be encouraged to interact with her (if only to exchange greetings). Listeners were encouraged to approach and then pause several feet on either side of her. Once Mary established eye contact, the listener would approach and begin conversing. This program encouraged staff to reinforce her use of a socially appropriate and conventional way of indicating a readiness and desire for interaction. It also provided natural opportunities for Mary to observe outcomes of her behavior (causality).

Perhaps the most relevant aspect of Mary's program was that it constructed contexts in which interactions with her could be assured. Teachers and others were pleased to accept Mary's now unambiguous bids for interaction. Once engaged, they were often likely to maintain conversations beyond mere greetings.

■□ NO ONE MODE OF COMMUNICATION IS ALWAYS PREFERABLE TO ANOTHER

One particular mode of communication may or may not be more effective than another depending on (1) the particular context, (2) the nature of the message, (3) the listeners' familiarity with the student (shared experiences), and (4) the listeners' relative familiarity with different modes of communication as used by the particular student.

In the early days of augmentative communication, it was generally felt prudent to opt for unaided modes of communication (e.g., signing) whenever possible (Shane & Bashir, 1980; Owens & House, 1984). This was particularly true for students who were ambulatory, in that too many problems arose transporting and caring for aided systems.

Over time, it was recognized that students with large repertoires of sign were often in the company of others who were unfamiliar with this mode of communication. Compounding the problem was that many of these students were taught modifications of standard signs. In some cases, the modified signs departed so drastically from the standard forms that persons familiar with sign were no more effective communicating with these students than those who were not.

Next, some clinicians and educators began concluding that unaided systems, particularly signing, were poor alternatives for students in light of the limited prospective audience for which this mode could be used. Classmates who had been encouraged to learn signs to communicate more effectively with nonspeaking students in their classes were then encouraged to ignore signs and redirect students to aided modes of communicating the same content.

Signing will always be of value to some students as one of several modes of communication. Signs that are highly transparent (i.e., able to be interpreted by laypersons) are particularly useful, as they require little or no listener training. Less transparent signs are also useful, especially with family members and others who are knowledgable of the mode and familiar with the student. Even modified signs are of use as highly efficient methods of communicating with a limited number of people. **The crucial point is not to avoid a particular mode of communication, but to instead offer multiple modes of communication that complement one another.**

We would not consider instructing nondisabled students to communicate through one mode alone, avoiding the use of pointing, gesturing, facial expressions, picture use, writing, computer, drawing, and so forth. Imagine a classroom in which the teacher asks a question and children are required to avoid all modes of communication other than the preferred mode: oral. Rather than a sea of raised hands, each indicating a desire to be called on, the teacher would be confronted with a cacaphony of voices. It makes no more instructional sense to impose such demands on students with disabilities.

Rather than actively discouraging one mode relative to another (i.e., mode devaluation), such as redirecting a child to sign when attempting to point or to indicate a symbol on a communication device when attempting to talk, it may be more useful for students to view the natural consequences of their mode selections. If a student uses a mode that results in an ambiguous message, there is a breakdown in communication. **Given an inclusive environment and a true desire to communicate, students and listeners can work together to identify optimal modes.**

■ TEACH COMMUNICATIVE BEHAVIORS THAT WILL BE EFFECTIVE WITH A RANGE OF LISTENERS

If we are to promote students' participation in a variety of environments and with a wide range of people, it is critical that their methods of communicating be easily recognizable. **If the time, complexity, ambiguity, and/or effort associated with a particular method of communication is too great, people are discouraged from interacting with the student.** The earlier example of Kevin and the Unicolor Binary Visual Encoding Board illustrates this point.

Judgments of system choice should be based not only on the perceived communication needs of the student, but the needs and abilities of listeners as well. This point is illustrated in the following cases of John and Pam.

> John indicated that he was finished eating by pushing his tray off of the table. Staff would encircle John, hoping to anticipate the moment he was finished, and then snatch his tray before it hit the ground. It was recommended that a piece of dison (a non-slip surface) in the shape of an "X" be placed on the table in front of John's tray. John was encouraged to signal classmates that he was done by pushing his tray to the "X," to facilitate tray removal.
>
> Over time, the dison was removed and John conveyed this same message by pushing his tray forward a few inches. Classmates and others were encouraged to consistently respond to John to reinforce the communicative value of this more socially acceptable indicator.

John's program served many purposes. One, it offered a more socially appropriate means of indicating that he was finished eating and needed help leaving the table. Perhaps more importantly, however, this revised method of communicating made John more likable to his teacher and aide and less intimidating to his classmates.

Pam, a third grader, was reported by teachers to have great difficulty making transitions from one activity to the next. They, along with Pam's classmates, held their breath as each activity wound down in anticipation of an outburst by Pam (screaming, kicking, clutching the materials she had been using, and so forth).

Pam's teachers were encouraged to provide clear cues that an activity was ending (e.g., remove their own materials first). In response to these cues from the teacher and modeling by classmates, Pam cleared her work space, too. A schedule board was developed to provide Pam clear cues about the sequence of classes and activities. After clearing her work area, Pam flipped a picture in her schedule that corresponded to the activity now completed. The following picture cued her as to where she belonged next (this was supported by teacher directions and modeling by classmates).

The solutions introduced with John and Pam shared three important characteristics: They were simple for the students and their listeners, and thus required minimal instruction; they required students and listeners to do things that were already familiar to them, and they corresponded to the task in which each student experienced problems. In addition, the behaviors targeted for instruction were ones that a broad range of listeners could interpret without difficulty. The latter point is addressed below as a 10th intervention principle (see Table 5–1).

■□ AVOID REPLACING ONE IDIOSYNCRATIC MODE OF COMMUNICATION WITH ANOTHER

The form and methods of communication that students use to communicate are of no consequence unless their behavior achieves what they set out to accomplish (e.g., request an object or action, comment, state, greet, direct another's attention, play, and so forth). Thus, it may be effective to encourage a student to smile to indicate "yes." However, problems would arise if the student used this or an indistinguishable response to also indicate, "I am bored," "I am tired," "please play with me," "I want to go out," "I want to stay inside," and so forth. Alternate means of expressing these different messages would be necessary to avoid misunderstandings and breakdowns in conversation.

■□ CHANGES IN COMMUNICATION SYSTEMS CAN ONLY ENHANCE COMMUNICATION WHEN STUDENTS PARTICIPATE IN CLASSROOMS AND OTHER SETTINGS THAT FOSTER INTERACTION

Like all children and youths, students with severe disabilities need opportunities to act on and be acted upon by others. Where the quality of these interactions is lacking (as perceived by these students and others in their environment), the need for augmentative and alternative communication (AAC) becomes both clear and desirable.

Similarly, when children's limitations with respect to communication restrict settings and experiences they are afforded, we can talk about the need for intervention. However, resulting programs must be motivated by concerns about the quality of students' lives (new experiences and opportunities which may be possible for the student) and not mundane changes in various esoteric measures of communication performance (e.g., length of messages, frequency of communication, and so forth).

The cases of Mathew, Todd, and Josie illustrate the role of the environment in fostering communication.

Matthew was a 4th grade student who exhibited great difficulties with communication. Much of his spontaneous language consisted of echolalic responses, comments that had no logical relationship to the conversation at hand, and repeating the same old information over and over, day after day.

In assessing Matthew's communication, his SLP was struck by the apparently limited opportunities he had to engage in novel experiences with classmates and others in or out of school. During the day, most of Matthew's direct instruction was carried out by an aide. His goals were always different from classmates', and often required different materials and settings to implement. Although much of his school day was spent in proximity to his classmates, they had little in common with one another.

According to his parents, much of Matt's life outside of school revolved around his home and yard. Opportunities to participate in group functions, soccer leagues, city-sponsored events, and so forth were limited. When he did attend, it was always with family members who served as buffers between Matt and others. Matthew's life changed dramatically following a school field trip aboard the sailboat of a classmate.

During and following the trip, Matthew's language and communication appeared to explode. He was eager to exchange feelings with others, comment about the trip, and answer others' questions, and so forth. He relished this rare occasion that had resulted in a set of shared experiences with classmates. He now had things to talk about that were of mutual interest to others. In addition, he had novel information to share with others who did not accompany him on the trip.

The SLP, Matt's parents, and other team members re-evaluated his communication program. To that point, the focus had been on skills such as increasing his use of appropriate language, encouraging him to maintain topics of conversation, and providing novel information to listeners. It was agreed that communication could not be addressed effectively unless and until Matt had people to interact with and things to talk about. Efforts by team members shifted to identifying activities at school and in his community in which Matt could begin to participate.

Staff reported that Matt's language improved dramatically soon after he began going to more places. He had things to talk about; novel information to share with others who were interested in what he had to say. A journal/scrapbook was introduced and transported by Matt between school and home. Several times a week, photos and other remembrances (e.g., ticket stubs, napkins from restaurants, portions of class projects) were included in his book as a means of stimulating conversations between Matt and others.

Todd used an electronic communication aid with voice output to augment his pre-existing repertoire of vocalizations and gestures. One day, I had the opportunity to observe him during science class. While his classmates worked on their group's experiment, Todd (in a wheelchair) was unable to reach the table on which the experiment was being conducted. Also, his classmates were unaware that while they stood around the table, he could not see past them.

Although Todd was an accepted member of the class, situations such as this arose regularly. Interestingly, one "communication" goal for Todd was to encourage him to request attention from others. Yet, despite appearing to want to participate in the group project, he was seemingly unable to alert others to his plight (then request that they move out of his way).

Earlier we noted that students may fail to demonstrate skills during formal instruction, despite reports that these same behaviors are evident under more natural conditions. Todd illustrated the converse situation, where students are unable to use skills functionally despite exhibiting these skills instructionally.

In this particular case, Todd's aide acted immediately. She took his hand, physically prompted him to tap the leg of the child who was blocking his view, then retreated a few feet away. Todd's classmate turned around, appraised the situation, apologized for being in Todd's way, then wheeled him around the table to an improved vantage point. As such situations occurred at other times of the day, the aide and Todd's classmates were asked to provide similar assistance to Todd. These events became the new instructional contexts in which requesting attention was targeted.

The need for and success of this particular aspect of Todd's program was contingent on classmates' acceptance of Todd and their understanding of how and why it was important that he participate in activities with them. In Chapter 2, we suggested ways of developing students' educational programs. One aspect of this process involves parties (the student, parents, teachers, classmates) identifying their respective roles in the student's educational process.

When students find themselves in situations in which teachers and classmates do not understand why they are there, it is unlikely that they will be afforded opportunities to participate. While educational goals have merit (with respect to their content), perhaps more relevant in the long run is the extent to which such goals provide a context for interactions between students. These points are illustrated by Josie and her class.

> Josie's classmates were aware that it was important for her teacher to ask her yes/no questions frequently to probe her comprehension of class material. Following each question, a classmate commented, "Okay, Josie, yes (raising and then dropping their right hand), or no (doing the same, but with their left hand). Which one is it?" This mode of communication, offered by a classmate spontaneously and inconspicuously, was acted on by Josie and her teacher. This enabled her to respond to the teacher's questions and allowed classmates to observe Josie's ability.

■□ COMMUNICATION SHOULD BE A TOOL FOR INTERACTION AND NOT SIMPLY AN ATTRACTIVE PROP

Years of attempts to augment students' methods of communication have demonstrated that although youngsters can "master" various electronic and nonelectronic modes of communication, these new competencies do not necessarily engender any meaningful changes in their daily lives (Calculator, 1988; Calculator & Dollaghan, 1982; Calculator & Luchko, 1983). The introduction of technology must be accompanied by efforts to appraise corresponding functional outcomes. Otherwise, technology may provide nothing more than attractive props, rather than tools for promoting interaction and inclusion.

Blockberger, Armstrong, O'Connor, and Freeman (1993) examine 4th grade children's attitudes toward a student who they observed (on videotape) using three different AAC techniques: aided electronic (a voice output communication aid—the ACS Epson HX-20 with Real Voice), aided nonelectronic (a communication board depicting letters of the alphabet), and unaided (signed English, fingerspelling, and vocal-verbal approximations). The children were asked to think about the student in the videotape as they completed The Chedoke-McMaster Attitudes Toward Children With Handicaps (CATCH) Scale (Rosenbaum, Armstrong, & King, 1986), a standardized measure of attitudes.

The CATCH consists of 36 positively and negatively worded statements. Items assess children's cognitive understanding of children with disabilities (e.g., "Handicapped children feel sorry for themselves," "Handicapped children like to play," "Handicapped children don't like to make friends"), their affective response to these children (e.g, "I would be happy to have a handicapped child for a special friend," "I would be pleased if a handicapped child invited me to his house," "I would feel good doing a school project with a handicapped child"), and their behavioral intentions toward children with disabilities (e.g., "I would talk to a handicapped child I didn't know," "In class I wouldn't sit next to a handicapped child," "I would invite a handicapped child to my birthday party"). The cognitive component examines others' beliefs about students with disabilities. The affective component assesses emotional feelings associated with these beliefs. Finally, the behavioral relates to others' ways of acting (or readiness to act) on their beliefs (Triandis, 1971).

Blockberger et al. (1993) find no significant differences in children's attitudes associated with the student's using the three different AAC techniques. Positive attitudes were related more to the sex of the respondents (females exhibited more positive attitudes) and their previous amount of experience with people with disabilities.

These findings indicated that access to technology (in this case an AAC aid with speech output) will not, in itself, result in improving children's attitudes towards students with severe disabilities. To the contrary, Cavalier (1987) proposes that one unforeseen outcome of providing access to technology may be accentuating the degree to which students differ from their classmates. An electronic communication aid is an ever-present cue to others that the student is in some way different.

Unlike Blockberger et al., Gorenflo & Gorenflo (1991) find that the attitudes of undergraduate students toward a nonspeaking 22-year-old college student grew more favorable as the sophistication of his AAC system increased (from unaided, to the use of an alphabet board, to a computer-based voice output communication aid). The fact that this latter finding contradicts Blockberger et al. is not surprising in light of evidence that attitudes appear to change from childhood to adulthood (Ryan, 1981).

The instrument that Gorenflo and Gorenflo (1991) used to assess attitudes, the Attitudes Toward Nonspeaking Persons Scale (ATNP), was designed (and validated) by these investigators for this study. The 29 items fell into two categories: general evaluation of the nonspeaking individual (e.g., "This person is not intelligent," "This person would be successful in a job," "This person should expect to lead a normal life") and an interactive/affective component (e.g., "I would feel uncomfortable with this person," "I would study [for a class] with this person," "I would help this person with a task such as purchasing something").

Gorenflo and Gorenflo (1991) also find that attitudes were more positive when the undergraduates had factual information about the student's physical disability (how cerebral palsy effected his ability to walk, talk, and so forth), social activities (hobbies and preferred activities [movies, reading, computers, and camping]), and his academic/employment status (the student had recently received his Bachelor of Science degree and had been previously employed by IBM).

An investigation by Bedrosian, Hoag, Calculator, and Molineux (1992) suggests that personal information about a particular student may be more relevant than general information about a population. SLPs with AAC training and experience were found to rate the communicative abilities of a nonspeaking adult less favorably than laypersons who had minimal experience with people with severe disabilities and minimal knowledge of AAC. Also, SLPs viewed the nonspeaking individual (an actor who posed as an adult with cerebral palsy) as more communicatively competent when his messages consisted of phrases rather than one-word utterances. For laypersons, message length was not as important a factor in judging communicative ability.

■□ ASSESSING OUTCOMES OF COMMUNICATION SUPPORTS

Changes in attitude constitute one of many methods (summarized in Table 5–3) of evaluating the effectiveness of attempts to promote inclusion through changes in communication programming (or, conversely, to promote communication by facilitating inclusion). Procedures cited in Table 5–3 reflect a philosophy of viewing communication as inseparable from inclusion and participation in regular school activities. The practicing SLP may find these measures depart significantly from more traditional indices of communication progress such as frequency of initiations, percentage of messages that are successful, average length of messages, number of symbols on a communication board, number of signs in an expressive repertoire, and so forth.

TABLE 5–3
Indications that communication supports are promoting inclusion

---

1. More positive attitudes by teachers, classmates, and others as measured by attitudinal surveys such as the Attitudes Toward Nonspeaking Persons Scale [ATNP] (Gorenflo & Gorenflo,1991): The Chedoke-McMaster Attitudes Toward Children With Handicaps [CATCH] (Rosenbaum, Armstrong, & King, 1986; Blockberger, Armstrong, O'Connor, & Freeman, 1993); and a questionnaire developed by Bedrosian, Hoag, Calculator, & Molineux (1992).

2. Teacher reports that more children offer assistance to the student during regularly scheduled classroom activities.

3. Classmates report that the students are more fun to be around.

4. Students are spending more time in the regular classroom, rather than being taken out of the classroom.

5. Students are participating more in the regular curriculum (as opposed to a personalized curriculum).

6. Students demonstrate increased use of positive social behaviors (e.g., approaching classmates, smiling, responding to questions, asking for and responding to others' requests for assistance) with concomitant decreases in socially undesirable behaviors (e.g.,

(continued)

TABLE 5–3
(continued)

---

hitting, spitting, self-abuse, and so forth). The Teacher Skill Checklist (McGinnis & Goldstein, 1984), described later, may be particularly useful in this respect.

7. Adaptive equipment (including AAC aids) is usually accessible.
8. Students are assuming a more active role in daily activities (e.g., what they eat, how they dress, where and with whom they play, where and with whom they do their schoolwork). This outcome depends greatly on teachers' and others' ability and willingness to offer students opportunities to make choices and indicate preferences.
9. Increased involvement in after-school activities.
10. Decreased need for one-to-one staffing (for assistance), with increased availability of informal and less intrusive supports from classmates and others.
11. Indications of enhanced status and acceptance by classmates, using sociometric ratings (e.g., Asher & Taylor, 1981) Classmates might be asked:
    "What three children would you most/least like to play with?"
    "What three children would you most/least like to work with?"
    "Which three children would you most/least like to sit next to you?"
    A point can be registered each time the students' name is mentioned, with comparisons made at diffferent times during the school year.
12. Indications of enhanced status and acceptance by classmates, using semantic differentials (e.g., Lass, Ruscello, & Lakawicz). Here, teachers, classmates and others use a Likert-type scale to indicate the extent to which various adjectives, often presented as polar opposites (e.g., pleasant-unpleasant, dependent-independent, caring-uncaring, friendly-unfriendly) describe a particular student.

■◻ SUMMARY

In this chapter we have cast communication into the broader perspectives of inclusive schooling and participation in regular classrooms. Communication demands pervade the curriculum, from specific skills associated with a classroom assignment to negotiating one's turns on a swing. The extent to which students are included relates to their abilities to meet these and associated communication challenges. SLPs can enlist the support of teachers, classmates, parents and others to provide settings that value students and the experiences they are willing to share with the rest of us. In doing so, they can not only have an impact on communication but, more importantly, on the quality of *everyone's* life at school, and beyond (the subject of Chapter 6).

■□ REFERENCES

Asher, S., & Taylor, A. (1981). Social outcomes of mainstreaming: Sociometric assessment and beyond. *Exceptional Education Quarterly, 1*, 13–40.

Bedrosian, J., Hoag, L., Calculator, S., & Molineux, B. (1992). Variables influencing perceptions of the communicative competence of an adult augmentative and alternative communication system user. *Journal of Speech and Hearing Research, 35*, 1105–1113.

Blockberger, S., Armstrong, R., O'Connor, A., & Freeman, R. (1993). Children's attitudes toward a nonspeaking child using various augmentative and alternative communication techniques. *Augmentative and Alternative Communication, 9*, 243–250.

Calculator, S. (1988). Promoting the acquisition and generalization of conversational skills by individuals with severe handicaps. *Augmentative and Alternative Communication, 4*, 94–103.

Calculator, S., & Dollaghan, C. (1982). The use of communication boards in a residential setting. *Journal of Speech and Hearing Disorders, 14*, 281–287.

Calculator, S., & Luchko, C. (1983). Evaluating the effectiveness of a communication board training program. *Journal of Speech and Hearing Disorders, 48*, 185–192.

Cavalier, A. (1987). The application of technology in the classroom and workplace: Unvoiced premises and ethical issues. In A. Gartner and T. Joe (Eds.), *Images of the disabled, disabled images.* New York: Praeger.

Ferguson, D. (1992, July). Is communication really the point? Some thoughts on where we've been and where we might want to go. A paper prepared for the *Second National Symposium on Effective Communication for Children and Youth with Severe Disabilities: A Vision for the Future.* McLean, VA: Interstate Research Associates.

Glennen, S., & Calculator, S. (1985). Training functional communication board use: A pragmatic approach. *Augmentative and Alternative Communication, 1*, 134–142.

Gorenflo, C., & Gorenflo, D. (1991). The effects of information and augmentative communication technique on attitudes toward nonspeaking individuals. *Journal of Speech and Hearing Research, 34*, 19–26.

Haring, N. (1988). A technology for generalization. In N. Haring (Ed.), *Generalization for students with severe handicaps: Strategies and solutions* (pp. 5–11). Seattle: University of Washington Press.

Jorgensen, C. (1992). Natural supports in inclusive schools: Curricular and teaching strategies. In J. Nisbet (Ed.), *Natural supports in school, at work, and in the community for people with severe disabilities* (pp. 179–215). Baltimore: Paul H. Brookes.

Kangas, K., & Lloyd, L. (1988). Early cognitive skills as prerequisites to augmentative and alternative communication use: What are we waiting for? *Augmentative and Alternative Communication, 4,* 211–221.

Lass, N., Ruscello, D., & Lakawicz, J. (1988). Listeners' perceptions of nonspeech characteristics of normal and dysarthric children. *Journal of Communication Disorders, 21,* 385–391.

Locke, P., & Mirenda, P. (1992). Roles and responsibilities of special education teachers serving on teams delivering AAC services. *AAC, 8,* 200–214.

McGinnis, E., & Goldstein, A. (1984). *Skillstreaming the elementary school child: A guide for teaching prosocial skills.* Champaign, IL: Research Press.

Mirenda, P., & Calculator, S. (1993). Enhancing curricula design. *Clinics in Communication Disorders, 3,* 43–58.

Owens, R., & House, L. (1984). Decision making processes in augmentative communication. *Journal of Speech and Hearing Disorders, 49,* 16–25.

Reichle, J., Feeley, K., & Johnston, S. (1993). Communication intervention for persons with severe and profound disabilities. *Clinics in Communication Disorders, 3,* 7–30.

Reichle, J., & Karlan, G. (1985). The selection of an augmentative system of communication intervention: A critique of decision rules. *Journal of the Association for Persons with Severe Handicaps, 10,* 146–156.

Rosenbaum, P., Armstrong, R., & King, S. (1986). Children's attitudes toward disabled peers: A self-report measure. *Journal of Pediatric Psychiatry, 11,* 517–530.

Ryan, K. (1981). Developmental differences in reactions to the physically disabled. *Human Development, 24,* 240–256.

Shane, H., & Bashir, T. (1980). Election criteria for the adoption of an augmentative communication system: Preliminary considerations. *Journal of Speech and Hearing Disorders, 45,* 408–414.

Triandis, J. (1971). *Attitude and attitude change.* New York: John Wiley and Sons.

6

Transitions to Adult Living: Promoting Natural Supports and Self-Determination

Laurie E. Powers and Jo-Ann Sowers

■☐ INTRODUCTION

Adolescence is typically a time for expanding personal independence, preparing for employment, post secondary education, and

The preparation of this manuscript was supported, in part, by Grant #H158K20006 from the US Department of Education, Office of Special Education and Rehabilitative Services and, in part, through the New Hampshire Natural Supports Project funded by the Department of Health and Human Services and the Department of Labor. No official endorsement should be implied, nor does this paper necessarily reflect the opinions or policies of any of these grant agencies.

community living, as well as developing new relationships with peers and community members. Each of these activities is essential if youth are to prepare for their quickly emerging adult roles, responsibilities, and privileges. Successful transition from adolescent to young adult roles is, in many cases, a natural and spontaneous process that becomes increasingly important to most teenagers as they move closer to graduation from high school (Larson & Kleiber, 1993).

For adolescents with disabilities, however, this process is often not so natural. Cognitive, physical, and health restrictions pose challenges to teenagers' efforts to live their lives as typically and independently as their peers without disabilities. However, the greatest impact on the future quality of life of teenagers with disabilities is the nature of educational and adult services available to them. During the last two decades, much attention has been directed by school and adult service programs toward identifying and implementing strategies to overcome barriers and promote successful transitions for students and young adults with disabilities. Through this process and, in conjunction with major shifts in societal views toward disability, the definition of "successful transition," itself, has undergone much evolution. This chapter provides an overview of the evolution of transition philosophy and services, describes emerging initiatives that emphasize natural supports and self-determination as critical factors for successful transition, and discusses the role of communication specialists in facilitating empowered and naturally supported transitions to adulthood for students with disabilities.

■□ EVOLUTION OF TRANSITION PREPARATION FOR STUDENTS WITH DISABILITIES

The purpose of school for typical students is to prepare them for adult life. School programs and curricula for these students are designed to teach students information and skills that will allow them to work and live successfully in society. As the demands and expectations of society evolve, school programs attempt to change to reflect these new expectations. For example, in response to the increasingly widespread use of computers in the workplace and every day life, schools have responded by teaching computer courses and incorporating computers throughout the curricula.

The goal of school programs for students with disabilities is also to prepare them for adult life and reflects societies' expectations for the type of life that these students will live. The nature of school programs provided to students with disabilities has evolved during the past two decades, reflecting dramatic changes in the expectations for the types of lives that they can and should lead as adults.

Preparation for Sheltered Living

Until the early 1980s, it was assumed that persons with disabilities, especially those with significant disabilities, could not work in regular businesses. This belief was based on the assumption that a person could work in regular businesses only if the individual had all of the skills and abilities to obtain, learn, and maintain a job in the same fashion as a person who did not have a disability. Consequently, a system of employment services was devised to teach these skills. Day habilitation programs were designed to teach "prevocational" skills, such as color identification, matching to sample, size and shape discriminations, letter and number identification, and basic living skills, such as shoe tying and tooth brushing. When all of these were mastered, a person could then "graduate" to a sheltered workshop.

SCHOOL AND ADULT SERVICES:
TRADITIONAL APPROACHES
CASE DESCRIPTIONS

In 1979, Jamie was 16 and entering high school. Jamie experienced significant cognitive disabilities and was unable to speak. Jamie's parents were told that she would continue to attend a self-contained classroom. However, she would spend several hours
(continued)

---

a day in one part of the classroom that had been set up as a sheltered workshop program. There she would learn pre-vocational skills including sorting (she would be given different size screws and taught to sort them into bins based on size) and basic manipulations such as threading nuts on bolts and taking them apart. Classroom instruction would be provided in basic skills such as identifying colors and numbers and self-care skills such as shoe tying and hair brushing. On Tuesday and Thursday, the class would go to the gym where they would be instructed by an adaptive P.E. teacher who would teach games to develop basic coordination abilities, such as dodge ball and races that required the student to go around obstacles set up in the gym. One day a week, a communication specialist would work with Jamie to teach her to use sign language.

Also during 1979, Patrick who was 23 years old and who had aged-out of the same program as Jamie, attended a day habilitation program 6 hours a day. At the program, Patrick performed the same type of prevocational skills as Jamie. Once a week everyone in the program went to the Easter Seals Society pool to swim. A SLP worked with Patrick once a week to teach him to point to pictures on a communication board. Patrick lived in a facility with 20 other persons with similar disabilities. Once a month, the facility took Patrick and several other "residents" into town for dinner and a movie.

In a sheltered workshop, "clients" typically spent part of the day working on subcontracted work brought in from a community business, typically involving assembly and packaging tasks. Most sheltered workshops also provided classroom instruction in academics and work-related topics such as job seeking and social skills. When a person was able to work independently and had learned all of the skills taught at the workshop, the individual was considered ready for job placement. At such a juncture, the work-shop staff would typically provide the individual with assistance in locating a position, but little other support in learning or keeping the job.

At that time it was also assumed that persons could live in their own apartment or home only if they could do so independently. A person with a disability who needed living support and did not live with family only had the option of living in a residential facility with other individuals who required similar types and levels of support. The facility might be a nursing home or a facility specifically for persons with disabilities. Residential facilities typically "housed" 10 to 30 individuals, with the goal of being to provide custodial care and supervision in the most efficient manner possible.

During that era it was also assumed that friendships could only be developed among people with disabilities and that separate activities for their recreational pursuits were needed. The popularity of Special Olympics and other disability specific recreational programs were an outgrowth of this assumption.

School programs reflected the adult service system philosophy and approaches of the times. Because it was assumed that most students with severe disabilities would enter day habilitation and residential programs, the schools focused on teaching those prevocational skills and basic self-care skills the students would perform in those environments. Rather than preparing students to transition from school to adult life, schools were preparing them for their transition from one program to yet another.

Emergence of Community-based Support Programs

In the early 1980s the traditional assumptions for people with disabilities and their place in society began to change. The realization that "get ready" models of employment and residential services did not work well was a major impetus to making these changes. Even after decades in a work activity center, sheltered workshop, or residential program, few individuals "graduated" to real jobs, real homes, or real lives. Through a number of demonstration and research efforts, it was also found that when a person with disabilities was provided the opportunity to work or live in a community setting and provided with training in the functional skills required in that settings, the individual achieved a level of independence previously not thought possible. Finally, there was a growing philosophical belief in the rights of individuals with disabilities to participate in and experience typical and regular lives. In response to these new perspectives, the focus on adult programs began to shift from one of preparation to one of providing support to individuals in situations that were as typical as possible of those in which adults without disabilities worked, lived, and participated.

CURRENT SCHOOL AND ADULT SERVICE APPROACHES CASE DESCRIPTIONS

Steve's day program adopted a supported employment approach. A job was found for him in central supply in a local hospital. His job was to put together three kinds of supply kits from different items. There were about 10 other employees who worked in the area. Steve's job coach remained with him for about 2 months. The job coach did an excellent job training Steve to perform his work. She devised a set schedule for him to follow-he would arrive at work, go straight to his work stations, and stay on-task until designated break times. The job coach arranged with the supervisors to remove any variations from his task schedule because this might cause confusion for Steve. Even though his co-workers had the option of going to break at different times depending on the amount of work available, she arranged for Steve to go to breaks at the same time each day, again to avoid confusion. Steve liked his job during these first 2 months-he liked earning more money than he had ever earned before and he liked all of the individual attention that he got from his job coach. After 2 months he had learned his job, was able to keep up with production and his job coach began to spend less time with him. At this time, Steve started to feel lonely and bored.

His co-workers were nice enough to him—they said "hi" to him in the morning; however, he really didn't know any of them and rarely interacted with them. Because Steve had a difficult time talking and being understood, his co-workers felt uncomfortable talking with him. In addition, he was self-conscious about how he spoke and he really didn't know what to say to them anyway. The few times he took a break with his co-workers, he sat there and didn't say anything.

To prepare for a job similar to Steve's, Jennifer began going to community work experience sites and learning to use the community when she was 15. By the time she was 17, Jennifer spent most of her day outside of the school building. Her special education teachers included transition planning in her IEP meetings. The teacher invited the vocational rehabilitation (VR) counselors and developmental disabilities (DD) case manager to the meetings. These professionals made sure that Jennifer was signed up for Social Security benefits when she was 18 years old. The VR counselor explained that her agency would pay a supported employment agency to place and train Jennifer and fund any adaptive devices that she may need at the job site, including a communication device. The DD case manager said that his agency would pay a supported employment agency to provide ongoing support to Jennifer.
However, he explained that unlike school there was no entitlement to adult services; his agency had a limited amount of money to serve a growing waiting list and people had to wait 2 or 3 years after they left school before their name came to the top of the waiting list. The VR counselor also explained that she could not pay for Jennifer to be placed on a job unless the DD agency had money to pay a supported employment for the ongoing support that Jennifer would probably need on the job. The special education teacher told them that it wouldn't be appropriate for the school to place her on a job unless it was likely that there would be

(continued)

> money for this ongoing support. However, they did get Jennifer signed up for VR just in case there would be money from DD and they put her on the DD supported employment waiting list. The case manager also informed Jennifer and her parents that the waiting list for group home services is so long that people typically wait 5 years before they get to the top of the list.

Without question, the advent of supported employment most profoundly reflected the evolution of thinking in the 1980s. Supported employment is based on the belief that all persons regardless of the nature and extent of their disability should have the opportunity to work in a regular business and that the role of employment services is to provide whatever support is needed to enable an individual to work in a real business in the community. A number of supported employment approaches emerged as the means to provide this support (Bellamy, Rhodes, Mank, & Albin, 1988; Rusch, 1986; Sowers, Jenkins, & Powers, 1988; Sowers, Thompson, & Connis, 1979; Wehman, 1981). Using the individual placement model, a job is found for a person that is suited to his or her current skills and abilities and a staff person provides training (job coaching) at the work setting for several weeks or months until the employee is able to perform the job duties independently. Using a crew or enclave approach, a group (eight or fewer as required by supported employment funding requirement) work under the supervision of a program staff supervisor at a company or companies. These group models have typically been used with individuals who are believed to not be capable of working "independently" and will need ongoing support. Today, through supported employment, close to 100,000 individuals with disabilities, including those with the most severe disabilities are working in community businesses (Sowers & Powers, 1991).

During the 1980s, there was also an attempt to provide more "homelike" living opportunities for persons with disabilities. During this time many of these people moved to small group homes (typically for five persons). Unlike earlier facilities that were institutional structures typically located in remote areas, family-style homes were purchased or built in residential areas. Attempts were also made to provide greater opportunities for participation in community leisure activities.

The adult service system evolution to supported employment, small group homes, and greater community presence had a tremendous impact on school programs. For the first time, there was a sense that students with disabilities really did have a future and that schools had an important role to play in preparing them for this future. During this time, the concept of transition began to gain prominence and was conceptualized as a three-component process. The first component was planning and preparation provided by the school program beginning when a student was 14 or 15. The second component provided program supports and assistance to individuals after they left the schools. The third component was coordination between the schools and adult service programs to ensure students moved successfully from one system of supports to another. The new approach used by schools to prepare students for this transition was derived from the belief that, if the goal for students is to work and live in their communities, then the focus of their program should be spent learning to work in community settings and developing functional living skills. With this is mind, schools were encouraged to have high school-aged students spend the majority of their time at work experience sites in community businesses, performing activities such as going to grocery stores to learn to shop and restaurants to learn how to order and pay for meals, and learning to cross streets and ride city buses. Schools were encouraged to introduce this functional curricula as early as middle school, with increasing time spent out of the school building and continuing until school services ceased (typically at 21 or 22, depending on the state).

At this point, students transitioned from services provided by the school to an adult vocational service provider. If a student had been placed into a job by a school job coach, the adult staff took over the training or ongoing follow-up support. If the student was not working in a paid job, the adult program had responsibility for placement. However, this transition only occurred if there was funding available from the state developmental disabilities agency to pay for the services. Additionally, if the student wished to leave home, a group home program was selected. Again, this occurred only if there was funding from the state agency to pay the group home program.

Shortcomings of Traditional Approaches

It is clear that supported employment, small group home programs, and community-based functional curricula for students with
disabilities represent a significant improvement over prior approaches. However, Steve and Jennifer's situations illustrate some
of the problems that the current approaches pose for students and
their families. At the very heart of these problems is their reliance
on staff-provided supports and lack of consumer self-direction. As
supported employment is currently practiced, program staff take
prime responsibility for determining the type of job in which a
person will be placed and for finding the job, with consumers and
families having at best, only minimal input and involvement in this
process. Program staff also take all responsibility for training and
support because it is assumed that regular supervisors and co-
workers do not have the ability or capacity to do this.

Several difficulties have arisen from this staff-reliant approach.
First, using the individual placement approach, it is hoped that the
supported employee will be able to maintain his or her performance when the job coach leaves the job site. However, because
the job coach typically provides all the training with little or no
involvement of the regular supervisor or co-workers, many supported employees become dependent on the job coach and their
performance does not maintain when the job coach leaves the
business. Second, it was hoped that by working in regular businesses, people with disabilities would have the opportunity to interact socially with non disabled employees and develop relationships
with them. Unfortunately, research and experience has shown that
the actual extent to which this has occurred for most supported
employees is minimal. The typical time and opportunity for developing relationships with co-workers for new employees occurs
during the first few weeks and months on the job, when co-workers are assisting the person to learn the job and how to fit in at
the worksite. Because the job coach takes responsibility for training the supported employee, the opportunities for co-workers to
get to know the individual during this critical initial period at the
site are limited. Individuals working in group approaches (i.e.
enclaves and crews) who receive ongoing support from program
staff have had particularly low levels of social interactions with
their co-workers without disabilities. Finally, the heavy reliance on
having program staff provide all of the placement, training, and support assistance is very expensive. The long waiting list for services

and the continued use of group models (which are less expensive than individual placements) are two unfortunate results.

With regard to group homes, the extent to which individuals living in these homes participate in community life, have networks of friends and acquaintances outside the homes, and lead normal and typical home lives is disappointing. These results can be attributed to a number of factors. Group homes, no matter how well run, are still "programs" with a need for rules, policies and regulations that often are considered more important than the needs and desires of the individuals who live there. The fact that five individuals reside together in a program sends a clear message to the individuals, to their families, and to the community that these individuals are different and need to be treated differently and supported only by paid experts.

With the implementation of functional curriculum, students with severe disabilities are leaving school much better prepared for adult life and work than when they spent their day in self-contained classes or segregated schools learning developmental and prevocational skills. However, the actual impact on these students' lives has been much less than expected. For example, Sowers (1983) found that although students were learning and performing functional skills in the community through their school program, very few participated in community life or activities outside of school. She also found that few students had formed friendships or acquaintances with non disabled peers. Additionally, a commonly heard concern of supported employment agencies is that, even though students have had work training and experiences through their school program, they are highly dependent and have difficulty interacting and socializing with co-workers. Agencies and families also express concern that young adults have difficulty making decisions and don't demonstrate "motivation" in adult settings.

■ EMERGING INITIATIVES IN FACILITATING TRANSITION

In response to the problems and issues discussed above, the field of disability services is beginning to evolve new approaches to promote participation in adult life. Two of the most significant emerging movements involve utilizing natural supports and promoting consumer self-determination.

Natural Supports

The Natural supports movement derives from the growing realization that if the goal is really for people with disabilities to live and work in fully included and typical ways, then we can only reach that goal by using approaches that are fully inclusive and typical (Nisbet, 1992). The naturally supported employment approach attempts to use processes that are like those used by persons who are non disabled to find, learn, and keep jobs and to empower individuals with disabilities and their families, friends, businesses, and co-workers to take the lead in this process. Young, non disabled persons seeking jobs typically get input from family and friends about the types of jobs to seek and often gain assistance getting a job through family and friend connections. Individuals with disabilities utilize their natural circles of support when job seeking and the role of the supported employment agency is to help bring together and empower the members of the circle.

NEW NATURAL SUPPORTS APPROACHES

Dave attended school in a district that was particularly progressive and had initiated a fully inclusive program for all students a year after he entered high school. During his first year, Dave was assigned a functional program. He spent most of his day out of the school at work experience sites and learning community functional skills. Although Dave enjoyed the program, he didn't feel like a high school student like his older sister who spent her day at school. Dave belonged to Special Olympics and went to practice once a week. He also had a friend from his class over once in a while.

The following year, Dave began taking regular classes with the help of an inclusion facilitator. The inclusion facilitator helped the class teachers to modify the curricula so that Dave could learn and participate in the class. Taking regular classes was scary for Dave and his parents weren't sure that it was right for him. However, after a few months

Dave felt for the first time that he was really a high school student who belonged at the school. He began making friends with a couple of students in his class, began going to football games and dances, and even joined the Pep Club. To get some vocational experience Dave enrolled in an automobile mechanics vocational education class, which met two periods daily. Dave had always been interested in cars and one day hoped to work around cars in some capacity. Although he wasn't able to learn the more sophisticated aspects of car repair, Dave learned how to help to change oil and tires and he specialized in car detailing.

At the end of his senior year, Dave graduated with his classmates. The transition specialist at the school spoke with several of the vocational education teachers Dave had in school and got the names of several businesses in town which focused on cars. The transition specialist asked the teachers to write Dave a letter of recommendation and she contacted them about a job for him. A part-time job was found for him at a car detailing shop in town. The transition specialist arranged for the businesses to receive on the job training funds from the Job Training Council and she provided suggestions to them about how to train Dave.

George, a young man not much older than Dave took the primary role as Dave's trainer. George was very easy-going and was well-liked by everyone who worked at the company. George had little difficulty training Dave; he figured out what Dave could and couldn't do and rearranged his tasks assignments and schedule accordingly. If he or Dave had a question about how to make something easier for Dave to learn, George asked the transition specialist.

Two day a week Dave attended a computer course at the Adult Learning Center. The tuition was paid for by vocational rehabilitation, because it was felt that by improving his computer skills,

(continued)

Dave's career potential could be expanded. In fact, his boss indicated that Dave might be able to help out entering customer information into the database maintained at work. An inclusion facilitator from the school worked with the Adult Learning Center's class instructor to make modifications in the curriculum and to provide other instructional assistance. The school also continued to provide support to Dave and his family, by teaching him community use skills. For example, the transition specialist helped Dave open a bank account and taught him how to deposit his checks from work. She also encouraged Dave's parents to allow him to go out after work with his co-workers to shoot pool on Friday nights and to go to the local car races.

After about 6 months at his job, Steve was having so many problems on the job that he was fired. Luckily, in the interim, the supported employment program learned about a new approach called naturally supported employment. Using this approach, they spent a lot of time really finding out the type of work situation in which Steve would be most motivated to do well.

They discovered that Steve had always dreamed of working in an office building and in a situation where he could wear a coat and tie to work each day. His brother, who he greatly admired, worked in an office and dressed up every day, so Steve thought a real job was one like that. In fact, Steve's brother, an insurance agent, gave the supported employment agency a number of names of businesses in town where he knew people who might be willing to hire Steve. Through one of these contacts a job was found in an attorney's office for Steve, where he did photocopying, filing and other clerical support tasks. When talking with the head of the clerical pool at the law office, the supported employment made it clear that their role was to provide consultation and assistance to their staff about how to train and support Steve, not to provide the direct training and supervision. The supervisor identified a staff person experienced with all of the tasks Steve would do and who she thought would be a particularly good trainer. This staff person was asked to serve as Steve's mentor and primary trainer during the first few weeks on the job. The employment consultant worked with this staff person to identify how to organize the tasks for Steve and provided her with hints and suggestions about how to train him. This mentor was well-liked by the other co-workers and she was able to introduce Steve to them and help them feel comfortable interacting with him. Through this approach, Steve did not become dependent on the employment facilitator, but rather learned to work with his co-workers as a part of the natural team. In addition, he had the opportunity from the very beginning to get to know his co-workers and to socialize with them.

When a non disabled employee begins a new job, the individual typically receives training from supervisors and co-workers. In addition, supervisors and co-workers typically provide support to employees throughout their employment. Today, many large companies have developed employee assistance programs that provide help to employees on a wide range of issues including drug, cigarette, and alcohol addiction: literacy education; counseling for personal, family, and work problems, and skill training. Most companies also provide significant levels of informal support. For example, one survey of companies found that supervisors spent more than 2 hours weekly speaking with employees about personal problems. Experience reveals that in the typical company, co-workers help, support, and cooperate with each other in getting work done as well as responding to personal and work-related issues.

In the naturally supported employment approach, the role of the supported employment agency is to provide consultation and assistance to businesses to empower them to train and support the employee with the disability. The focus of the employment consultant or facilitator is not only on helping co-workers to train and support the employee to perform the job, but also assisting the employee to become fully and meaningfully integrated into the social and cultural fabric of the worksite.

In the realm of living arrangements, natural supports recognizes that if we want individuals to live normal lives, to be fully integrated into their communities, and to have meaningful friends and connections, then they must live in ways that non disabled people live. It is not typical for five unrelated roommates to live together, especially if the decision to live together was not their own and was made based on a physical or cognitive ability characteristic. Today, there is a growing movement to provide individuals, even those with the most significant disabilities, the opportunity to rent or even own their residence, to live alone or with a roommate of their choosing, and to hire the person who will provide them with assistance (Kline, 1992).

The implications of natural supports for school programs are enormous. Again applying the principle that if we want students with disabilities to be fully integrated into society and to lead the same types of lives as non disabled students, then they must be provided with the same types of experiences as these other students. Obtaining work experience and developing vocational skills is important for students with and without disabilities. The typical ways students without disabilities get this experience is through vocational education classes and after-school and summer jobs. Some schools have apprenticeship, internship, and work study programs for students, offer students the opportunity to get credit for participating in a business mentorship program, or require students to spend a certain number of hours each week doing community service. These types of experiences are valuable for all students and special educators should work with regular educators to implement these programs and to make them available to *all* students (Tashie & Schuh, 1992).

Students with disabilities should also spend most of their day in school, not in self-contained classrooms, but in regular classes, alongside their peers who are non disabled. By doing so, a clear message will be given to their peers, who will later be employers and co-workers, to families, and, most importantly, to the students themselves that they belong in society on an equal footing. Other important outcomes will also likely occur. These students' peers will learn to feel comfortable being and interacting with individuals with disabilities. Students with disabilities will also learn to feel comfortable being and interacting with individuals without disabilities and to learn critical social skills that can only be learned by practice, feedback, and exposure to daily modeling.

Students should also have the opportunity to learn functional independent living and community-use skills. However, these should be taught in the context in which these skills naturally occur. For example, rather than teaching a student to go grocery shopping as part of a school class, the school should encourage and assist the students' parent to have the student participate in and learn how to shop. The school may assist the parent by giving suggestions about ways the student could participate in shopping and, if needed, to actually accompany the parent and student on occasion to illustrate ways to include and instruct the student.

Typical, non disabled students graduate and leave school when they are 18 or 19 years of age. Students with disabilities should also graduate and leave school with their same-age peers. However, this does not necessarily imply that students give up the right to educational assistance at that time, but rather suggests that the type of assistance should change. The time between 19 and 21 is when schools, in coordination with adult service programs, can actively assist students to enter the adult world. Young adults who do not experience disabilities have a variety of options. They may choose to continue their education in college, obtain vocational training through a technical school, go to work, or do a combination of these activities.

Students with disabilities should have the same options open to them. Of course, the prospect of a student with a significant cognitive disability attending college seems to many more far-fetched than inclusion in regular classes in high school. It's useful to remember that 20 years ago, the idea of community-based employment for these same individuals seemed far-fetched to most people. Across the Nation increasing numbers of students are attending college classes and living in dorms. While still enrolled in high school a young woman named Angie took a horse technology class at the University of New Hampshire, and Lisa, who used facilitated communication, took an English literature class.

The division of vocational rehabilitation will pay college tuition if the courses taken will lead to a job. If the tuition can be paid by vocational rehabilitation, the family or student, then the school should provide any support or assistance the student may need while attending class. A few examples of assistance include sending an assistant to class for physical or other support, providing a teacher who can make suggestions about curriculum modification to a professor, or sending a communication special-ist to consult with professors about how the student will ask and answer questions in class.

A large number of young adults choose to enter the labor market when they leave high school and it is likely that this will be the option chosen by many students with significant disabili-ties. Given that, in many communities, inadequate funding is avail-able for supported employment services and an individual may not be able to get these services for several years after leaving school, it is critical that the schools put job placement at the top of the priority list for students. If a student can be assisted in finding a job and secured in this job through natural supports, then the individual may not have to sit home for several years, waiting for adult services-provided supported employment.

During the critical period when students are between 19 and 21 years of age, the school should also focus on helping connect them to other young adults and young adult community activities. While in high school, students take physical education. When they leave school, they may take an aerobics class or lift weights at a health club. While in high school, a student's friends are typically limited to other high school students. When students leave school, they begin to develop an expanded network of friends and ac-quaintances of other young adults. When students leave school they typically begin to think about moving out on their own or they remain at home with increasing amounts of freedom and responsibility for themselves (e.g. contributing to household bills). Again, students with disabilities should have the same opportu-nities as typical students and schools should assist them during the critical period of transition between the ages of 19 and 21.

Self-determination

Although they use feedback and support from others, adults with-out disabilities are primarily responsible for making their own decisions and actively pursuing their personal goals. Young adults without disabilities decide what kind of work they want to do, how far they're willing to travel to get to work, and what hours they're willing to work. They are responsible for getting to work on time, doing their best on the job, and making decisions about how best to spend their money. Most individuals typically rent or own their place of residence and, thus, have ultimate say over what goes on there (e.g., who comes and goes, who they live with, how it is decorated). Many people have individuals who come to their homes to help them (e.g., with housecleaning, yard maintenance), however they choose who these persons will be and they hire them. Most individuals also have the freedom to come and go in the community based on their personal schedules and desires, rather than being dependent on the availability and desires of the other members of the household or professional staff.

SELF-DETERMINATION APPROACH: CASE EXAMPLE

Susan was a junior in high school and enjoyed attending classes with her non disabled peers. One reason Susan enjoyed school was because she was able to select her classes and took major responsibility for developing her IEP. Each year, Susan had a series of meetings with her inclusion facilitator. They discussed Susan's dreams for the future and the facilitator assisted Susan to develop some short term goals consistent with her future plans. Susan then informally discussed her plans and annual goals with her parents and obtained their feedback and support.

When Susan was clear about her goals, she invited people important in her life to participate in a planning meeting that also functioned as her IEP. Susan led the meeting with prearranged assistance provided by the facilitator. Susan invited participants to describe the activities they had helped her to accomplish the prior year. Next, Susan shared her goals and asked each participant to present a plan for how the person could assist Susan to achieve each goal. A friend who attended indicated he would be willing to accompany Susan to the spa she wanted to join. The speech therapist offered to help Susan add some community-referenced words to her communication device. Her math teacher committed to

(continued)

assist Susan to learn how to balance her checkbook in association with Susan's goal to open up a checking account. Each commitment was recorded on Susan's IEP and procedures for Susan to monitor her progress on goals were noted.

Following graduation at 18, Susan continued to utilize a similar procedure to select goals, enlist the help of others to reach her goals, and monitor her progress. Eventually, Susan developed two different teams of people and recruited several individuals to support her; one team helped her find a job, another helped her move into an apartment, and a family friend assisted Susan in hiring her first personal assistant. A peer counselor from a local independent living program helped Susan to set goals and manage her supporters by reminding Susan of the strategies she could use in helping her to structure her plans; however Susan was in charge and fully responsible for her life.

Adults with disabilities should have these same opportunities for self-direction, optimal independence, and assumption of personal responsibility. Although family members and many professionals question if typical levels of self-determination are "realistic" for people with significant cognitive disabilities; once again, it is important to remember that just 15 years ago, most thought it unrealistic for people with disabilities to live and work in the community. During the mid 1980s, the question of whether it was possible for people with disabilities to succeed in the community was reframed to ask, "What supports would be necessary to enable a person to succeed in the community?" This reframing of the question enabled us to shift our focus to identifying and demonstrating innovative models to promote community living. A similar reframing process is essential for self-determination if we are to fully discover potential strategies for promoting consumer empowerment. The question addressed must be "What does it take?" rather than "Is it possible?"

Little attention has been focused directly on preparing students to assume responsibility for their own transition (Mitchell, 1988).

Even less attention has been directed to the development of specific student-directed strategies to enhance the self-determination of transitioning students who experience significant challenges. Exercise of self-determination is a critical facet of successful adult inclusion (Varela, 1986; Ward, 1988). Although the Independent Living Movement has done much to enhance the self-determination competence of adults with physical disabilities, it has had relatively minimal impact on school-age students and their parents, and, in particular, those students who experience cognitive disabilities.

The identification of skills and experiences that promote self-determination for youth with disabilities is the focus of increasing attention in education and rehabilitation. Although there is widespread agreement that self-determination is important for independence, adherence to traditional notions of special education and rehabilitation as "expert" professions, with special understanding of the needs of people with challenges remains, to some extent, antithetical to current notions of consumer empowerment and control. As a result, many interventions developed to enhance self-determination, continue to focus on identifying methods to encourage consumers to make decisions and attempt behaviors that professionals and parents believe are appropriate rather than facilitating truly consumer-directed choice and action. What is needed to actively promote consumer self-determination is the identification of methods that consumers can use to identify and achieve their goals and to manage supports provided by professionals, families, and others in their lives.

Approaches to promote self-determination must have as their centerpiece implicit and explicit support of youth as effective change agents in their lives, capable of exercising personal control and decision making. Furthermore, interventions should be designed for primary implementation by youth, with others acting as facilitators for youth expression of self-determination. Theory and research related to the development of self-determination (Bandura, 1986; Bednar, Wells, & Peterson, 1989) suggests that self-determination is influenced by several sources including (a) vicarious learning from observing others successfully demonstrating self-direction; (b) active, successfully participation in personally valued, ongoing activities that build competence; (c) verbal persuasion by others that reinforces capabilities; (d) physiologic feedback that reinforces perceptions of self-competence; and (e) successful use of strategies to productively manage frustration and failure. Building self-determination thus requires exposure to situations and supports that maximize these sources of influence. Current models (Powers, 1993) suggest three critical approaches for promoting self-determination.

Provide Opportunities for Successful Participation in Typical Experiences

If teenagers with disabilities are to develop greater independence and self-confidence, they need, foremost, to have access to environments that provide typical opportunities for youth to try new activities, build skills, take risks, assume responsibilities, form friendships, and learn strategies to productively manage frustration. For youth without challenges, these opportunities are typically provided through their experiences in school, with peers, and at home. Going to school with other youth from the neighborhood, doing home chores and earning privileges, shopping for popular clothing, and endlessly talking with friends on the phone are examples of typical experiences that provide many opportunities for teenagers to learn independence and responsibility. It is essential that teenagers with challenges have access to the same opportunities. Insisting that an adolescent be permitted to attend his or her neighborhood school, assigning family responsibilities, and providing transportation or other help to encourage involvement with peers are examples of important ways to provide such access. Because youth with disabilities will ultimately have and want to assume responsibility for their ongoing medical and personal care, it is also important that they have opportunities to train and supervise their school aides, perform self-care routines, schedule medical appointments, meet privately with their doctors, and gradually assume greater control over their medical care decisions.

Providing these opportunities is not easy in some cases: encouraging self-care may take extra time and disrupt routines, negotiating with service providers and professionals can be very frustrating, and encouraging independence may be scary, because some experiences don't work out and it's painful to watch a teenager fail or be rejected. Yet, there aren't many alternatives if youths with challenges are going to be adequately prepared to reach their potential for independence and feel like they can succeed in our typical world. Clearly, providing such opportunities requires commitment, support, and collaboration among youth, families, and professionals. Furthermore, the strategies families use to provide independence opportunities will differ and families must be supported in making choices that are consistent with their values and feasible to implement.

Assist Teenagers To Learn Skills for Managing Barriers

In most cases, teenagers learn "typical" independence skills in the context of participating in ordinary activities. However, to be successful and overcome atypical barriers, youth with disabilities may need to learn additional skills or approaches. One such skill is **goal setting**. A way to approach this is to assist teenagers to develop some ideas about what they want their futures to be like and identify some activities they are not doing or doing at less than optimal levels of independence that they could do more independently to work toward their future dreams. Most adolescents have dreams about working, going to college, having friends, and living on their own. Commonly related goals for adolescents and young adults include learning to manage money, exploring post high school educational and vocational options, planning recreational activities, and developing friendships and romantic relationships (Clark, Mack, & Pennington, 1988). As students identify these activities they can be encouraged to explore their personal goals and choose specific activities to engage in that are consistent with those goals. For instance, a youth who wants to make friends might choose to start talking to other students in the hall, invite someone to his or her home, or join a school club. As parents know, teenagers often resist choosing goals they believe are imposed by others. They tend to become most invested in goals that they think are relevant to their self-perceived needs. Typically, teenagers will be more likely to view goals as relevant if they pick them and see a connection between working on a current goal and reaching desired levels of future independence.

A second important skill is **problem solving**. Learning how to problem solve is particularly essential for teenagers with challenges who have to overcome many barriers to do ordinary activities. To assist teenagers to become good problem solvers involves teaching and modeling a basic approach they can use to figure out how to do activities *and* providing them with the support they require to successfully apply the approach to achieving their personal goals. When a student with a disability has difficulty performing an activity, it is normative for related service staff to be requested to apply their expertise to assist the student to perform the activity. Occupational therapists (OTs), physical therapists (PTs), or speech and language pathologists (SLPs) may observe the student attempt the activity, analyze the youth's difficulty, and suggest adaptive equipment or other strategies the student could use to do the activity.

Although this approach is often efficient and effective, it fails to provide youth with the experiences they need to learn to independently identify strategies they can use to perform activities. As such, it falls short of promoting youth independence and development of self-perceptions that they have the necessary capabilities to figure out how to successfully achieve outcomes in their lives. To address these needs, it is essential that related service staff use consultation opportunities to teach and model for youth methods they can use to figure out how to do activities. These methods might include assisting students to identify the steps they will have to perform to do activities, figure out in detail what is hard to do, and brainstorm potential solutions. When solutions are identified that involve selecting and ordering adaptive equipment, youth should also be introduced to equipment catalogues and taught how to order devices. By giving this information away to students, related service staff can significantly empower students with skills they will need to apply throughout their lives.

Students with significant cognitive challenges may have difficulty independently mastering problem solving however, they can still be assisted to learn the process and enlist the help of others to identify specific strategies they may be able to use. For instance, a student may learn to first identify what he or she wants to do and what's hard before asking for help. Instead of merely notifying a speech therapist that he or she can't use a communication device, a student can learn to communicate that he or she can't turn it on because the switch is too hard to press. Providing this information will assist the therapist to identify appropriate solutions, ensure that the student gets the right help, and promote the student's perceptions of personal control.

Another skill teenagers and young adults need to learn is **planning.** Effective planning is often a critical determinant of successful participation in activities for youth with disabilities. It is common for parents and school staff to plan activities for youth with disabilities. Yet, unless youth learn how to plan their activities they will forever be dependent on help from others. To help youth plan, they can be coached to create comprehensive "road maps" for performing their activities and complete preparation tasks to ensure their plans will be successful. For instance, a student who wants to make breakfast for him or herself may decide that one strategy he or she will use is to keep the cereal on a lower shelf of the cupboard. However, for the student to successfully use that strategy, he or she will have to prepare by asking family members to store the cereal on a lower shelf. Such negotiation with family members can be novel and intimidating for inexperienced teenagers and may require development of a script for what to say and opportunities for rehearsal. Assisting students to identify and complete these types of preparation tasks will enhance the potential for students to both successfully use the strategies they select and perceive that they are capable of managing their lives.

To be successful, teenagers with disabilities also have to develop expertise at **building and managing helping partnerships** with other people. Partnerships may need to be developed with friends, family, school staff, community agencies, and personal assistants. Partnership skills may include learning to identify who can be of assistance, enlisting support, demonstrating assertiveness, self-advocacy, and negotiation, and monitoring and managing help that is provided. For students with disabilities, the key to enhancing self-determination involves both maximizing independent performance of activities *and* skill at directing the help they receive from others. In reality, these keys to self-determination are not substantially different than those for youth without disabilities. We live in an interdependent world in which both engaging in independent activity and developing partnerships with others is essential for personal success. However, because they may have ongoing needs and are required to interface with complex service systems, youth with disabilities often have to develop additional expertise in enlisting and managing assistance from others.

In managing personal assistance, students often need to learn (a) recognition of accurate helping routines or specific behaviors performed by the student and his or her helper; (b) delivery of instructions to helpers; (c) strategies to stop helpers when they are providing incorrect help; and (d) strategies to thank helpers at the conclusion of routines. It is essential that school staff define their roles to include facilitating student acquisition of expert support management skills and provide opportunities for students to practice their skills in the context of managing their aides and IEP teams. Helping teenagers learn and practice partnership skills, including managing personal assistance, will promote self-determination and ensure that students are prepared to transition into an adult world in which they must be prepared to assume primary responsibility for working with others to achieve their goals.

Provide Support to Promote Self-determination

All of us require support from others to feel competent and achieve goals. Practical help, encouragement, and information are a few types of support that seem to be important for most people. Unfortunately, teenagers with disabilities tend to be provided with support that is inadvertently disempowering. Support provided to these teenagers tends to focus on their limitations or involves doing activities for them rather than providing support to enhance their abilities to make decisions and do activities as independently as possible. In contrast, empowering support might include providing information about choice options, giving encouragement and praise for trying, or delivering an occasional "kick in the pants" that forces assumption of important responsibilities or challenges a teenager to make active decisions about how much independence he or she really wants to strive towards. To facilitate enhancement of the self-determination of young adults, school and adult service staff must be willing to provide youth with access to information and experiences that will promote their decision making and convey confidence in their abilities to make effective judgments (Mitchell, 1988).

Talking openly with a teenager about the challenges of disability and helping him or her to identify strategies to manage problems is another important form of support. Many teenagers have important questions and concerns about their health or future disability, friendship, dating, and life after high school that they need acknowledged and discussed openly. Practical help is also essential and can be very empowering when provided in the context of a teenager choosing help and taking responsibility for managing it. Teenagers with challenges who don't have opportunity for contact with peers or successful adults with similar challenges may also find this form of support useful as they confront disability-related barriers and plan for the future.

Roles of Speech-Language Pathologists (SLPs)

In the previous sections, we offered a description of issues that typical adolescents encounter and experience when transitioning from school to adulthood. We also provided an overview of a new philosophy and set of approaches that attempts to ensure that students with disabilities make this transition in ways that are self-directed, typical and natural. These changes in secondary education and transition services for students imply critical changes for the role of professionals. In this section we will focus in particular on the role implications for SLPs.

Employment

It is obvious that communication is critical to any person's employment success. The actual performance of most jobs requires at least some degree of communication with co-workers (asking questions, giving information, answering questions). As we suggested, an important aspect of work is the opportunity to interact with and socialize with co-workers. SLPs should be prepared to provide consultation related to the type of communication strategies that will enable an individual to be successful and fully integrated at the business where she or he is employed. To do so, SLPs must gain an understanding of the world of work and the realities that operate there. Of course, the communication demands of each business and job are unique. An SLP can provide input and suggestions about how an individual can best communicate given the specific demands of the job and business. For example, Susan, who has cerebral palsy, worked at a credit union doing clerical support tasks. She photocopied, made membership packets, and typed and laminated new members cards. Susan was able to speak, but was somewhat difficult to understand. She had an electronic communication device that she kept on a lap board on her chair. While doing these tasks, her lap board had to be removed for her to access essential materials and machinery (typewriter, photocopier). Consequently when working, Susan did not have access to her communication device.

The employment facilitator, Susan, and the SLP discussed her situation. The SLP suggested that, while Susan was performing her tasks, she could attempt to communicate verbally with co-workers. To make this as easy as possible, the supervisor, Susan, and the SLP identified the types of things that Susan would need to communicate to co-workers as part of her job. The SLP also identified some key phrases that Susan might need to say while working (e.g., "I'm going to lunch" or "I need help") and coached her to say these as clearly as possible. Susan and the SLP also met informally with each co-worker. Susan said each of the key phrases, while the specialist indicated to the co-worker what she was saying. After listening to Susan say each phrase several times, the co-workers were able to understand her. The SLP also explained to each co-worker that Susan wanted colleagues to ask her to repeat something if they did not understand and that they should feel comfortable asking her to do so. Finally, Susan and the SLP showed each co-worker how her electronic device worked, as she would be using it during breaks when she could access it and would want to have extended social conversations with co-workers over coffee.

Community Living

When individuals with disabilities were expected to spend most of their time in segregated settings or receive constant supervision in community settings, issues of communication were relatively simple. Now that there is a real desire to enable individuals to have full community access in ways that utilize natural supports, the manner in which individuals will communicate in these settings becomes both paramount and complex. An SLP must be willing and able to step out into the community with the individual to help the person to determine the demands of each environment in which the individual wishes and needs to communicate and to identify the best strategies for doing so. Perhaps the most important point that a SLP must understand is that each and every situation is unique and, thus, the manner in which the individual can best communicate in each may be different.

Devin, who is unable to speak, wanted to be able to live in his own apartment and enjoy the community independently. It was clear that communication would be one of the major challenges he would face. How would he make phone calls? How would he order food in a restaurant? How would he ask for help in a store or on the street if he needed it? How could he tell the ticket taker at the movie theater what show he wanted to see? The SLP who consulted with Devin understood that his method of communication would need to be tailored to each situation. Devin had a portable electronic communication device that was useful for him to use when he could place it on a table and there was sufficient time for him to type out what he needed to say. However, this was not possible in many circumstances, such as when asking for help on the street or telling a ticket taker what movie he wanted to see.

The SLP and Devin identified each situation in which he might need or want to communicate and problem-solved communication strategies he would use. For example, in the movie theater, they decided that Devin would type out the name of the movie on a typewriter at home and present the paper to the ticket taker. To enable Devin to order food at his favorite fast food Mexican restaurant, the SLP typed up the menu on a small card that Devin carried in his back pack. When he went to the restaurant, Devin pointed to appropriate words on his card to communicate which food items he wanted.

Friendship

Communication is a tool for developing interpersonal skills, self-understanding, and learning developmental norms and expectations for behavior-all critical elements for building and maintaining friendships (Hill, 1983). As is the case with promoting communication in employment and community settings, facilitating communication with friends also requires detailed attention to context. However, context in this case often includes both the demands of the setting in which a person wants to communicate with friends (walking down the street, sitting in a restaurant, etc.) and specific demands for communication as a function of the nature of the friendship a person has with whomever he or she is spending time. For instance, the conversation that might take place between two close friends at a ball game might sound very different than a conversation between two casual acquaintances or two people on a date at the same game. To add further complexity to this issue, it's important to remember that individuals, particularly adolescents and young adults interact with friends idiosyncratically. Learning to talk to friends is a real challenge for all young people and figuring out how to "fit in" often requires detailed consideration of variables such as the topics typically discussed by friends and expressions used.

John, a junior in high school who recently began attending regular classes, decided he wanted to start eating lunch with students from his classes. John had an electronic communicator that worked pretty well when he had time to spell out the words and the people he spoke to were close enough to hear his electronic voice or read his screen. However, at lunch John didn't have much time and his device was difficult to position so he could both eat and use it so other students could see the screen. John also had difficulty getting the attention of the other students and explaining to them how to talk with him. John explained this situation to his SLP and they agreed that observing John at lunch might help his SLP to help John figure out strategies he could use to talk to other students. The following day, the SLP nonchalantly observed John at lunch. It was clear that, in addition to the challenges John identified, he also appeared uncomfortable and didn't attempt to join in on the conversation.

During their next meeting, John and his SLP agreed that he needed (a) a way to quickly explain to the other students how to talk to him, (b) some conversation starters and nonverbal strategies to show he was listening and fitting in during conversations, (c) an alternative to his electronic aid that was quicker to use and could be easily positioned for different students to see. They decided to begin by both programming into his device and writing on a card information about how to talk to John. The few sentences explained that John wanted to talk and used either his aid or a communication book to speak. To start a conversation, John would tap the student on the arm or look at the student and make a sound. If he had a specific thing to say, John may have already typed it into his device and be able to just push a key or two to make the aid say and spell his message. If he wanted to join in on a conversation, he would spell words and point to pictures in his communication book. In response, he needed the students to listen to or read what he said. John also emphasized that he understood them and they didn't have to do anything special to talk back to him.

John and his SLP then developed a communication book that included typical words John might want to use with other teenagers. John decided to include some vulgar and slang expressions that were normally used by the students. They also added these words to his device. Next, John and his SLP identified some conversation starters to program into his aid and add to his book. That way, John could use his aid or book to get a conversation going quickly. In addition to some standard conversation starters, the specialist encouraged John to think ahead about topics he and others might want to discuss over lunch. Sports was a frequent topic, and John decided he would program ahead of time into his device or write in an erasable section of his book, questions or reactions to recent football or basketball games he saw on TV. That gave John novel topics to discuss at lunch with his friends.

To help John look more comfortable at lunch, he and his SLP also rehearsed methods for John to attend nonverbally. He learned to make eye contact, laugh when others laughed, and start out by just saying "hi." They also decided that because it took extra time for John to communicate, he would join into conversations by using phrases whenever possible. With practice and coaching, John became good at communicating efficiently and his friends showed greater interest in what he was saying. As time passed, he was able to begin communicating longer phrases and sentences because he had their interest and they became comfortable with talking to him. From time to time, John and his SLP debriefed about how John was doing with lunch-time conversation and the specialist also assisted John to adapt his strategies to communicate with friends in restaurants in the community. Eventually, they wrote out instructions that John could show his friends to train them to help him add new words to his device. This activity turned out to be a lot of fun for his friends, helped to normalize their interactions, and reduced John's reliance on his language specialist.

■ SUMMARY

Much evolution has occurred in societal and professional views about the potential for people with disabilities to live, work, and participate in post secondary education in typical settings side-by-side with people who do not experience disabilities. There is now a strong and growing commitment to inclusion, the promotion of natural interpersonal ties between people, regardless of challenge, and consumer empowerment. Concurrent with our evolution in thinking has come significant developments in the design of strategies to promote typical transitions for young people with disabilities, and both school programs and adult providers are increasingly integrating these methodologies into their transition support services.

SLPs have a unique opportunity to contribute to these efforts. In conjunction with current trends toward expanding the role of schools to focus on the enhancement of functional skills in community settings, there is immense potential to target intervention efforts to assist students to build and expand their access to, and use of, natural supports. Furthermore, such interventions can be consciously designed in partnership with youth to integrate strategies that promote their development and demonstration of skills essential for self-determination. The extent to which SLPs and other support professionals integrate such strategies into their work with students will be a key determinant of their abilities to truly promote the capacities of students with disabilities to transition into self-directed, naturally supported lives.

■◻ REFERENCES

Bandura, A. (1986). *Social foundation of thought and action. A social cognitive theory.* New York: Prentice-Hall.

Bednar, R. L., Wells, M. G., & Peterson, S. R. (1989). *Self-esteem: Paradoxes and innovations in clinical theory and practice.* Washington, DC: American Psychological Association.

Bellamy, G. T., Rhodes, L. E., Mank, D. M., & Albin, J. M. (1988). *Supported employment: A community implementation guide.* Baltimore: Paul H. Brookes.

Clark, F. A., Mack, W., & Pennington, V. (1988). Transition needs assessment of severely disabled high school students and their parents and teachers. *The Occupational Therapy Journal of Research, 8*(6), 3323–3344.

Hill, J. (1983). Early Adolescence: A research agenda. *Journal of Early Adolescence, 3,* 1–21.

Klein, J. (1992). Get Me the Hell Out of Here: Supporting People with Disabilities to Live in Their Own Homes. In Jan Nisbet, *Natural Supports in School, at Work, and in the Community for People with Severe Disabilities* (p. 300). Baltimore, Maryland: Paul H. Brookes.

Larson, R., & Kleiber, D. (1993). Daily experiences of adolescents. In P. H. Tolan & B. J. Cohler (Eds.). *Handbook of clinical research and practice with adolescents* (pp. 124–126). New York: Wiley.

Mitchell, B. (1988). Who Chooses? *Transition Summary, 5.* Washington, DC: National Center for Handicapped Children and Youth.

Nisbet, J. (1992). *Natural Supports in School, at Work, and in the Community for People with Severe Disabilities.* Baltimore, MD: Paul H. Brooks.

Powers, L. E. (1993). Promoting adolescent independence and self-determination. Association for the Care of Children's Health. *Family-Centered Care Network, 10*(4).

Rusch, F. R. (Ed.). (1986). *Competitive employment issues and strategies.* Baltimore: Paul H. Brookes.

Sowers, J. (1983). *Validation of the weekly activity interview (WAI): An instrument designed to measure the lifestyle of severely handicapped secondary-aged students.* Unpublished doctoral dissertation, University of Oregon, Eugene.

Sowers, J., Jenkins, C., & Powers, L. (1988). The training and employment of persons with physical disabilities. In R. Gaylord-Ross (Ed.),

Vocational education for persons with special needs. Palo Alto, CA: Mayfield Publishing Co.

Sowers, J., & Powers, L. (1991). *Vocational preparation and employment of students with physical and multiple disabilities.* Baltimore: Paul H. Brookes.

Sowers, J., Thompson, L. E., & Connis, R. T. (1979). The food service vocational training program: A model for training and placement of the mentally retarded. In G. T. Bellamy, G. O'Connor, & O. C. Karan (Eds.), *Vocational rehabilitation of severely handicapped persons: Contemporary strategies.* Baltimore: University Park Press.

Tashie, C. & Schuh, M. (1992). Why not community-based instruction. In C. Jorgensen (Ed.), *Equity and Excellence* (newsletter), (pp. 15–17). Durham, University of New Hampshire, Institute on Disability.

Varela, R.A. (1986). Risks, rules and resources: Self-advocacy and the parameters of decision-making. In J. A. Summers (Ed.), *The right to grow up. An introduction to adults with developmental disabilities*, (pp. 245–254). Baltimore, MD: Paul H. Brookes.

Ward, M. (1988). The many facets of self-determination. *Transition Summary,* 5. Washington, DC: National Center for Handicapped Children and Youth.

Wehman, P. (1981). *Competitive employment: New horizons for severely disabled individuals.* Baltimore: Paul H. Brookes Publishing Co.

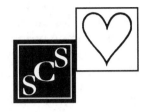

Epilogue

Beth Dixon

■ WITH EVERY ENDING THERE IS A NEW BEGINNING

Andrew started 5th grade this fall. Why does "5th" sound so much older than "4th"? No year ever begins as smoothly as the one before ended. There is a new team of players. He has a new teacher and three new aides who assist him throughout the day.

No one really knows who the real Andrew is yet. The time it takes to introduce Andrew and his many talents and quirks to others is very frustrating for me. The challenge for us is to try to figure out a way to make each new beginning less stressful. We're working on it!

I had been questioning the wisdom of "attaching" an adult to a child for several years. It seems only normal that if an adult is constantly there, a dependency will arise from both sides. This seems especially true for a child who can smile and con anyone into doing things for him that he should be doing more independently!

At our IEP meeting last spring, the team made a decision to have more people involved with Andrew, to decrease his dependency on his assistant. He has transitioned beautifully to so many people, but it hasn't helped the main problem—dependence on adults!

The other more significant problem with having Andrew "and company" is the time and opportunity it can take away from more typical kid-to-kid interactions. Ten and 11 year olds don't want an adult hanging around listening to their conversations and watching their every move. We, as adults, often create a larger problem than we begin with! Another challenge! Andrew's friends are comfortable assisting him when necessary and hanging out with him. We all need to learn to ask the kids for their input, and truly listen to their suggestions.

Dreams and Detours

Andrew, despite our concerns, is loving the 5th grade—even the homework! One dramatic change for our family this fall has been the absence of teenagers in our home. Our three older children are all in college and Andrew is adjusting better than I am to his being the "only" child. He has visited each of them in their dorm or apartment. He is very excited to see each one whenever they can make it home. When they leave, he settles in quickly to his new role. I think that when I figure out how to cook for three people instead of six, I will have mastered this stage of my journey!

Our vision for Andrew is very typical and the same vision we have for all of our children. We want him to be happy and healthy, to be loved and accepted for who he is, to have good friends, to have choices in his life, and the supports to make his choices possible. These choices will include whether to go to college or not, working at a job that he enjoys, deciding where he lives, who he lives with, and what he does in his free time for recreation and travel.

I know we are on the right road every time I walk into Conant School and hear so many kids say, "Hi, Andrew" and as an aside to me, "He's in my class." Every afternoon when I pick him up at the Boys and Girls Club after-school program, and it takes me 3 or 4 minutes to find him in the crowd , I am assured once again that, "separate" is not "equal." I know all is well on the social scene because right now there is an invitation to a birthday party for this Saturday afternoon sitting on our kitchen counter!

I am reminded often of one of my favorite quotes by Ursula K. LeGuin: "It is good to have an end to journey towards: But it is the journey that matters in the end." For Andrew, the journey has begun and we know the end we are traveling towards is more "typical" than "special." There may be road blocks along the way, but there are also detours. It is on these detours that we find beautiful places that we may otherwise have not encountered. I am sure that in the end, Andrew's journey will have mattered and made a difference in the lives of everyone he has met along the way.

The last 4 years have been the best so far for Andrew and our family. Real friendships have developed, changes in the attitudes of school personnel and the community are positive, and Andrew has grown socially, academically, and communicatively. He has taught everyone around him to avoid judging people by their label, to keep an open mind, have high expectations for everyone, and to value all people for their strengths. No, he isn't "fixed" and yes, he still has disabilities. He is still Andrew, my beautiful 10-year-old son!

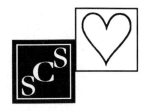

Index